55 ESSENTIAL BALANCE EXERCISES FOR SENIORS

A SIMPLE SENIOR-FRIENDLY GUIDE TO FALL PREVENTION, IMPROVING STRENGTH, STABILITY, POSTURE & LIVING A MORE INDEPENDENT LIFE

BRANDON LEE

FREE BONUS 90 DAY WALKING PROGRAM DOWNLOAD

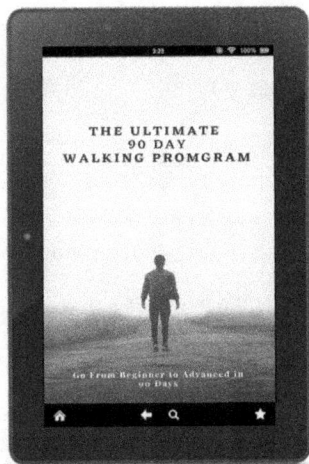

Before you begin this book, please take advantage of the **FREE** Bonus *"Ultimate 90 Day Walking Program"*. Inside this guide you will receive a day by day, week by week walking plan to help build cardiovascular capacity and increase lower body strength.

To receive your FREE Bonus "Ultimate 90 Day Walking Program" scan this QR code!

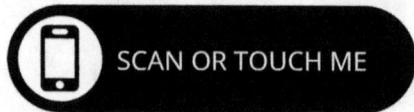

SCAN OR TOUCH ME

CONTENTS

INTRODUCTION

Did you know that 1 in 5 older adults suffer from balance issues globally? The risk of falling due to the imbalance in the elderly population is causing significant problems for seniors. You may feel frustrated if you have already enjoyed 50 summers of your life and now have difficulty walking or performing your activities of daily living independently.

Aging is a blessing and an unchangeable reality if we are lucky to do such. Our muscles become insufficient as we age, and the risk of falling due to weak muscles also increases significantly. All these issues are interconnected, and the single most efficient solution for every problem is "exercise." Many believe that strength training and balance exercises for the elderly are harmful. However, scientific research shows quite the opposite.

Why Are Balance Issues So Prevalent In Older Adults?

High-quality scientific literature has shown that the loss of muscle mass between 40-80 years of age is almost 30%-60%. That means the chances of muscle weakness and the resulting problems, imbalance ,and the lack of independent movement increase to nearly sixty percent in an 80-year-old adult. The issue can be more significant when an older adult suffers from other health conditions (e.g., diabetes, Parkinsonism, Alzheimer's disease, etc.).

One-third of the elderly population has been reported with multiple falls during a calendar year because of imbalance. The weak skeleton is a super-imposed issue, and the chances of fracture (or more severe injuries like brain concussion) are more prevalent in older adults suffering from balance issues.

The inability to move independently is also causing severe mental illnesses in older adults. The prevalence of depression in older adults who require assistance with their activities of daily living is 11.5% more than in those who don't have mobility issues. The confidence of older adults suffering from balance issues is also severely compromised, leading to a steep rise in the prevalence of social isolation and loneliness.

What Is The Most Effective Solution?

The good news is that all these issues are resolvable. You can easily prevent muscle weakness, the risk of falling, and balance problems with the help of a carefully catered exercise program. It is equally valid for those already suffering from these issues mentioned above to implement a customized exercise plan to enhance mobility and help boost confidence.

Balance exercises and strength training are cost-effective yet highly efficient ways to help prevent falling in older adults. Progressive strength training can increase muscular strength in older adults by increasing muscle mass and the brain's control over muscles. It directly improves the balance in the elderly and significantly reduces the fall risk. The importance of this book lies in achieving these exercise goals.

How Can This Book Help You?

I have written this book to help you overcome balance and strength issues by incorporating a carefully planned set of 55 exercises. This book will help you efficiently design your customized workout plan to target your personal needs. Remember that the improvement in balance and strength is a gradual process and should be targeted in a step-by-step fashion. Most online resources ignore this critical fact altogether, resulting in a catastrophe.

This book keeps the importance of gradual improvement in mind. Exercises for older adults should be cost-effective, easy to perform, and safe. You might be suffering from an illness that can further deteriorate your balance, so the prescribed exercises should cater to your specific needs; this ideal helps separate this book from others similar.

You will know the proper form of every exercise included in this book and the recommended exercise volume (no. of sets, repetitions, etc.). This book also provides information about the target muscles for each exercise. This knowledge is crucial to lay down the foundation of an efficient start, and you can track your improvements as you proceed to the more advanced levels.

Nothing Is Superior To The Professional Expertise

My grandparents raised me, and I saw them struggling with their daily activities. Their difficulties in performing their tasks independently and suffering from multiple falls motivated me to gain expertise in the art of elite-level personal training for seniors. It is not just a hobby for me; I have an emotional attachment to the cause.

I have been personally training senior adults for years, and the participants improvements from my specialized exercise programs has brought me much joy!

I didn't gain this knowledge overnight and have spent significant time collaborating with doctors from around the world and learning from highly authoritative scientific resources. I know the struggles of seniors in performing strength/balance exercises and appreciate the gradual improvements. Regaining balance and muscular strength take time, but it is worth it.

Knowledge is power; you must gain it before jumping into advanced steps. You must know balance, strength, posture, and mutual relevance. You must understand how an elderly body works and the best approach to become independent in your daily living activities.

Are you ready to age with confidence? Keep reading!

CHAPTER 1
THE BASICS OF BALANCE

The ability of the body to keep the center of mass above its support base is known as balance. Humans with a fully working balance system can easily detect their orientation with gravity and estimate the direction and speed of their movement. This ability allows them to adjust automatically to maintain posture and stability in various situations and activities. Balance is a critical sense that provides much-needed steadiness to our upright and moving bodies.

Sensorimotor control mechanisms establish and maintain balance. These mechanisms include sensory input from vision, touch, and the vestibular system (motion, equilibrium, spatial orientation); sensory integration; and motor output to the eyes and body muscles.

One or more of these components can be affected by injury, disease, certain medicines, or aging. Psychological elements may affect our sense of balance and the contribution of sensory information.

The balancing system has many connections with the brain. These connections show that the forces of motion we create and meet in the environment can affect various brain regions. These brain regions control vision, hearing, sleep, digestion, learning, and memory.

WHAT IS THE MECHANISM OF BALANCE?

Every sensory system has receptors outside the brain to gather information about the environment. The visual system, for example, detects visible light using light-sensitive receptors in the retina. The inner ear's balancing system is based on specialized motion-sensitive receptor cells.

Our central nervous system manages sensory information from other systems to provide appropriate muscular output to maintain a controlled, upright posture is referred to as postural control or balance. The primary sensory systems involved in posture regulation and balance are the visual, vestibular, and somatosensory systems.

Proper postural control is the ability to engage in a variety of static and dynamic activities, such as sitting, standing, walking, and running, while contracting the appropriate muscles for a controlled upright posture and making minor adjustments in response to changes in position and movement without the use of compensatory motions.

Unfortunately, all these interconnected systems become less efficient as we age. Diseases like Parkinsonism and diabetes can further deteriorate balance in older adults.

Balancing the body has two main functional goals:

· Postural orientation

· Equilibrium

The alignment and tone of the body are controlled by the postural orientation of gravity, the support surface, the visual environment, and internal references. Postural equilibrium is defined as the synchronization of sensorimotor methods to stabilize the body's center of mass during self-initiated and externally induced stimuli.

THE VISUAL SYSTEM

Because the visual system is the primary receiver of sensory information for maintaining the balance of the body, our postural stability improves as the visual environment improves.

There are two types of eye movements:

Gaze Stabilization:

The movements keep the image of a visual target focused on the eye's fovea when the head moves. The fovea is a slight depression in the rear side of our eyes. It is the center of the field of vision on the eye's retina. The retina is a thin layer of tissue covering our eyes within our eye socket.

Gaze Shifting:

The movements keep the image of a target focused on the eye's fovea when the visual target moves.

Gaze Stabilization

Two gaze stabilization mechanisms operate during head movement:

· The vestibulo-ocular system

· The optokinetic systems

Coordinated movements of eyes (also called conjugate movements) are required for good gaze stabilization. These are the movements in which both eyes move in the same direction.

Shifting Of the Gaze

Three gaze-shifting techniques are used to focus the image on the fovea.

1. **Smooth chase**

It is a visual tracking technique that uses the eyes to track the movement of a visual target. It allows us to stabilize the image of a moving target on or near the fovea. Pursuit eye movements are voluntary, smooth, continuous, conjugate eye movements whose velocity and the moving visual target determine the trajectory of our vision.

1. **Vergence**

It adjusts the angle between the two eyes to compensate for variations in visual target distance. The process through which the eye shifts focus from distant to near images is accommodation. The eyes converge (are pointed to the nose) while altering one's perspective from a distant object to a nearby object to keep the object's picture fixed on the foveae of the two eyes.

1. **Saccades**

These eye movement types consist of brief, jerky motions with a preset (between two fixed points) trajectory that leads the eyes toward a visual stimulus. The eye movements are made to bring an object of interest into vision.

THE VESTIBULAR SYSTEM

The Vestibular System is a part of the human body responsible for hearing. This system uses sensory orientation and weighs relevant sensory inputs to balance the body vertically in various sensory settings, such as standing on an inclined surface, on foam, or with their eyes closed.

The vestibular system also regulates the body's center of mass in static and dynamic postures (a person stands or walks on a beam) and stabilizes the head during postural movements when the person leans or tilts.

Inner Ear and Endolymph

While the inner ear is most commonly connected with hearing, it also serves as a center for equilibrium. It features a labyrinthine (complex and twisted) structure with fluid-filled tubes and ducts. Five balance receptors are strategically distributed throughout the labyrinth to detect various forms of movement.

Each balance receptor is a multicellular organ with long hair-like projections. When we move our heads, these so-called hair cells are activated when their projections are pushed in a particular direction by a fluid called endolymph.

When the head starts to move, the endolymph remains still at first. This results in a rapid relative endolymph migration in the opposite direction of the head. The hair cells that are aligned to detect that particular head movement are excited by this relative movement.

Endolymph and hair cells work together to accurately send a steady stream of information regarding head movement to the brain. The ability of the inner ear balancing organs to detect minute and significant head movements, rapid and slow, and in any direction, is impressive. The brain then organizes a set of balancing reflexes that regulate our muscles down to our toes.

On the other hand, these reflexes control our postural and eye muscles. These reflexes work together to stay upright with stable eyesight in a constantly changing and shifting physical environment.

Again, the irony of aging makes all these reflexes less efficient. The result is a potential fall risk because of progressive balance issues in the older population.

When we jog, why doesn't our eyesight bounce up and down?

The function of our incredibly delicate and responsive balancing system is to maintain our upright posture. It does, however, significantly impact our ability to control our eye movements. Walking or jogging causes our vision to become unstable due to the up-and-down motion.

Like footage from a hand-held camera, a simple jog along a flat route or a smooth road might result in unstable and wobbly photos. It can be uncomfortable and challenging to focus on stationary objects like trees when watching hand-held camera footage since they move too quickly.

Vestibulo-Ocular Reflex

Our visual field is surprisingly stable when we are exercising. This is due to the vestibulo-ocular reflex, which most of us take for granted.

The vestibulo-ocular reflex is one of the human body's fastest and most active reflexes. It uses the inner ear to detect head motions and generate compensating eye movements that are identical in magnitude but opposite in direction to the head motion. This subconscious, continual adjustment of eye location results in a steady visual field despite the severe head movement.

THE SOMATOSENSORY SYSTEM

The somatosensory system is a sophisticated network of sensory neurons and pathways that responds to changes on the body's surface or within. This system relays information from muscles and skin to the brain. It also aids in postural balance by relaying information about body position to the brain, which allows it to initiate the proper motor reaction or movement.

Mechanoreceptors are sensory receptors found in the spindles of muscles. They give information to the neurological system about the length and rate of contraction of muscles. This information indirectly helps the person differentiate between joint movement and position sense. Afferent feedback (that travels from muscles to our brain) from the muscle spindles produces appropriate reflexive and voluntary actions.

Because the upper neck region contains more muscle spindles, it connects to the visual and vestibular systems. An injury to the upper cervical (neck) region causes more sensorimotor dysfunction than the lower cervical region.

Summary of Balance Control Systems

The visual, vestibular, and somatosensory systems are part of a more extensive postural control system that works together to keep you balanced.

Good sensorimotor integration between the upper cervical spine, ocular, and vestibular regions leads to position stability. If there is a sensory mismatch, the central nervous system (CNS) cannot differentiate between accurate and inaccurate sensory information from one or more of these systems, resulting in instability, poor balance, and disruption in sensory input prediction timing.

If you suffer from this condition, you can have headaches, blurred vision, eye strain, and balance issues. When gazing up at the board and down at the desk during note-taking, you may have difficulties reading (horizontal deficits) and feel dizzy (vertical deficiencies). As the body tries to adjust to a loss of equilibrium, neck pain is expected due to increased muscular stiffness. Some older adults with balance issues report feeling lost and overwhelmed when driving in a new city, through tunnels, or pulling a grocery cart through the corridor.

What happens if the balance is off?

The prospect of abruptly losing a sense like eyesight or hearing is horrifying for many people (and correctly so), and losing your sense of balance would be similarly disastrous.

Initially, you would be unable to complete routine activities without falling over due to painful and scary dizziness. The worst symptoms will fade as you rely more heavily on other senses, such as eyesight. However, even a partial loss of the vestibulo-ocular reflex would require you to come to a complete stop and stand still every time you wish to recognize a face or check the price of a supermarket item.

We are entirely unaware that this graceful reflex demonstrates the excellent secret work the balancing system performs. It allows us to walk without tripping and provides a consistent and reliable picture of a constantly changing world.

FALLS ARE NOT FUNNY

After all, falling is a terrifying experience. The majority of individuals are aware that falls are dangerous for senior citizens.

According to the Centers for Disease Control and Prevention (CDC), one of every five falls results in a severe injury such as a broken bone or a concussion. The fear of falling can hurt an aging adult's quality of life and, unfortunately, can prevent them from being active and prospering.

Because the hazards of falling in seniors are so severe, many elders and family caregivers are interested to know about fall prevention. While it's impossible to prevent every fall, it's usually always possible to take steps to lessen the risk of a severe injury.

What causes a person to fall?

Regardless of who you are or your age, here's why you are more prone to falls:

Our ability to keep upright is not greater than a challenge to our balance or strength.

Put another way; we fall when we encounter an event that causes us to lose our equilibrium or strength. If our ability to stay upright is overwhelmed by this event, we will fall.

We have a strong ability to keep upright while we're youthful and healthy. As a result, if we trip, we can usually catch ourselves and recover before falling. However, muscular imbalance dramatically affects balance, making even a young person fall. If that same young person is weak or intoxicated, it will take much less force to disturb the balance resulting in a fall.

Another scenario that will limit the capacity of anyone to keep upright is illness or weakness. This is why hospital patients of all ages are prone to falling.

However, older folks often have various additional issues limiting their ability to stay on their feet. The falls in older individuals are usually invariably "multifactorial." This means that a fall, or a person's risk of falling, is frequently caused by a combination of variables.

There are three categories of fall risk variables to consider. I also find it helpful to categorize the factors into one of three groups:

1. **Health-related Problems**

Balance issues, weakness, chronic illnesses, visual issues, and drug side effects are all examples. They are unique to a single individual.

1. **Hazards by the environment**

In-house dangers (e.g., loose throw rugs), outdoor hazards (e.g., icy sidewalks), and dangerous footwear (e.g., high heels) are examples of these. Improper usage of a walker, cane, or other assistive device falls under this category.

1. **Triggers**

These are unexpected or infrequent events that jeopardize your balance or strength. It could be as simple as a strong dog pulling on a leash, or it could be something more severe like low blood sugar (hypoglycemia) in a person with diabetes.

It will most likely be difficult for you to compile a list of these criteria independently. Health-related factors, in particular, are frequently linked to medical issues. As a result, unless you've learned much about medicine, it can be challenging to sort them out appropriately.

Still, I advise older persons and their caregivers to consider fall risk factors since this can help them ask their doctors the right questions.

HOW TO PREVENT FALLS IN SENIORS

Trying to handle every single factor can be difficult. Slower reflexes, for example, are sometimes hard to reverse. Still, it's a good idea to read over them and try to spot a handful that are either simple to correct or might significantly reduce the chance of falling.

Here's what you can do to prevent yourself or your loved one from falling.

- Make a list of the elements influencing an older person's risk of falling.
- Determine the risk factors and triggers for recent or recurring falls.
- Determine which factors are the easiest to adjust or modify. Determining factors is partially about the component in question and partly about what my patient can change. (Stairs can be dangerous, but moving to a new home without stairs can be difficult.)
- Implement practical tactics to address fall risk variables that can be changed.

Tips for Finding your Balance

The following points can help you know about your postural balance.

- Figure out which leg, right or left, is your dominant side. To simplify the exercises, begin each repetition with your non-dominant side
- Maintain proper form and posture while in the exercise position.
- Fix your eyes on a fixed point straight ahead to keep the balance.
- If you're having trouble keeping your balance when standing, consider putting your feet a little further apart.
- Slightly bend your knees. This keeps your knees from overextending and gives you more stability.
- Try to distribute your weight equally between both feet. Take note of whether you tend to place more weight on one foot than the other or whether your weight shifts forward or backward.
- You might try closing one eye at a time, gazing up at the ceiling, or trying other arm positions as your balance improves.

Exercises To Prevent Falls and Improve Balance In Old Age

While it is impossible to prevent a fall completely, balance and strength training exercises can help lessen the chance of falling. These exercises can help you improve your balance and strength, which will help you avoid falling in the future.

Activities such as squatting, standing up from a chair, and walking may be complex or unsteady for older persons, increasing their risk of falling. The activities below are designed for people with a low risk of falling and who can stand independently without assistance. Before beginning any new exercises, consult your doctor or physical therapist, especially if you have poor balance.

BALANCE TRAINING

If your balance is shaky, try this set of exercises. Make sure you're accompanied by someone in case you lose your balance. Standing in a corner or having a kitchen counter nearby to grab if you start to lose your balance.

1. Feet apart

Stand with your feet shoulder-width apart and your eyes open for 10 seconds, gradually increasing to 30 seconds.

If you find yourself wobbling or reaching for the wall or counter a lot, keep practicing until you can do it without swaying or assistance. Move on to the next exercise once you can hold this position for 30 seconds.

2. Feet together

Stand with your feet together and your eyes open for 10 seconds, gradually increasing to 30 seconds.

Move on to the next exercise once you've completed this for 30 seconds with minimal wobbling or support.

3. One foot

Stand on one foot with your eyes open for 10 seconds, gradually increasing to 30 seconds. Shift your weight to the other foot.

4. Closed eyes

If you can safely complete the prior three exercises with minimal assistance, try each with your eyes closed. Hold for 10 seconds at a time, gradually increasing to 30 seconds.

The goal for each exercise is to hold the position for 10 seconds and then move to 30 seconds, five repetitions per leg on the one-foot exercise, and two times per day. It's critical to discuss fall prevention with your doctor or physical therapist. Talk to your doctor about any drugs you're taking and any adjustments you've made to your workout program.

Of course, this is not the complete list of exercises to help you overcome your balance issues. As we proceed with the following chapters, we will cover the 55 most beneficial exercises that can help you perform your activities of daily living with more confidence.

CHAPTER 2
START WITH A STRETCH

Are you ready to hit the gym or the dance floor... or at the very least go for a daily walk now that you've heard about all the benefits of fitness as you age? The only issue is that your joints or muscles refuse to cooperate. Is it too late to get in shape?

According to the American College of Sports Medicine, flexibility (the range of motion of joint and soft tissue) declines with age and physical inactivity. Flexibility allows us to improve our range of motion, performing everyday chores such as bending down to tie our shoes or quickly reaching for a dish on a shelf.

Over time, inactivity can cause your muscles, tendons, and ligaments to shorten. Stretching can help develop your flexibility and prepare your body for action at any age. But don't forget that cardiovascular fitness and strength are equally crucial as you become older. Stretching exercises for seniors can enhance flexibility and quickness, lowering the energy required to execute a movement and, most importantly, preventing injury.

STRETCHING EXERCISES TO INCLUDE IN YOUR WORKOUT

Physical activity is essential for a better overall quality of life, especially for seniors. Exercise keeps our bones strong, backs straighter, and can help postpone the onset of diseases like diabetes, relieves arthritis pain, improves our mood and mental health, and is crucial in preventing falls. It's never too late to incorporate exercise into your everyday routine!

If you already exercise daily, you must stretch your muscles appropriately. Stretching loosens your joints by stimulating the fluids within them, which helps to prevent friction-related damage. Stretching also assists in lengthening your muscles, which are more susceptible to injury when they are short or tight. You'll see immediate effects when you incorporate stretching into your training program.

Stretching Techniques that Work

Follow these guidelines to incorporate flexibility exercises into your fitness routine:

- **Take your time**

Slowly ease yourself into the stretch. A slight pulling sensation should be felt in your muscles, but it should not be uncomfortable. A stabbing pain indicates that you've gone too far. If you're new to stretching exercises, keep in mind that your muscles will take some time to loosen up.

Relax and take a deep breath. When stretching, never hold your breath. Breathe into the exercise. Gently push yourself a little further with each breath.

- **Keep an eye on your spine.**

Keep an eye on your spine's position. Allowing it to curve too far can make you prone to harm. Maintain flexibility in your back and joints by never locking them into place.

- **Do Not Bounce**

Don't try to extend your reach by bouncing into a stretch. To ease into the stretch, utilize steady motions rather than jerking movements since the faster movements might cause the muscles to tighten instead of loosening!

- **Keep that stretch going.**

Allow at least 30 seconds in each stretching posture to allow the muscle to lengthen appropriately. Breathe in, exhale out, and try stretching a little further the next time.

Suppose you're just getting started with a fitness program. In that case, you should incorporate stretching into your warm-up and cooldown to help with any stiffness that may arise from your activity. Always consult your doctor before beginning any new physical activity to determine the best course of action for your specific health needs.

BENEFITS OF STRETCHING IN SENIORS

Maintaining movement might be challenging for many older people. Our muscles and joints weaken as we age, and our range of motion decreases. Stretching improves the quality of life and promotes healthy aging by developing and maintaining strength, enhancing flexibility, and increasing circulation and blood flow.

1. Stretching helps with arthritis and low back pain

The most prevalent causes of lower back discomfort in older persons are arthritis and spinal stenosis. The most prevalent type of arthritis is osteoarthritis, characterized by the slow deterioration of cartilage between the facet joints. The discomfort in the lower back usually comes and goes, but osteoarthritis can eventually lead to sciatica. Osteoarthritis of the low back is prevalent, but arthritis of the hips, knees, neck, fingers, and toes is also common.

The narrowing of the bone channel occupied by the spinal nerves or cord is known as spinal stenosis. Sciatica is when the spinal nerves become compressed, causing tingling, weakness, and numbness in the low back, buttocks, and legs.

While osteoarthritis and spinal stenosis are unavoidable consequences of aging, the pain they cause can be alleviated with stretching exercises.

Seniors benefit from regular stretching because it improves flexibility, range of motion, and elasticity, which helps to reduce stiffness in the affected joints. It's understandable that stretching and moving these joints might be difficult and uncomfortable. Warming stiff muscles with a heat pack before stretching and cooling down muscles with an ice pack following exercise can help lessen discomfort and reduce swelling. You may also think about stretching with the help of stretching equipment or another person.

2. Improved Physical Performance

Becoming more flexible can make daily chores like lifting, bending, twisting, and participating in other repetitive actions easier and less tiring.

3. Stretching lowers the chance of falling

Falling is a big issue for seniors, especially those aged 65 and up. Every year, one out of three older individuals falls, resulting in 2.5 million people requiring treatment in emergency rooms.

Lack of flexibility can lead to a loss of balance, resulting in falls and injuries. Regular stretching will help you maintain a decent range of motion and avoid accidents that could result in mobility loss.

Regular bouts of stretching are beneficial to balance and stability and prevent falls. Fall prevention in older persons requires increased flexibility in the hamstrings, quadriceps, lower back, and increased hip joint mobility.

4. Stretching aids in the correction of improper posture

The water content of the connective tissues, such as ligaments and tendons, declines as we age, resulting in decreased flexibility. The tightening of ligaments and tendons added with years of sitting, bent over at a desk, tend to cause poor posture in the chest and shoulders. A forward head position, rounded shoulders, upper back, and forward pressing hips are all signs of poor posture.

The inherent S-curvature of our spine compresses. Pain in the lower back and between the shoulder blades may result. Since stretching improves flexibility, it assists in releasing stiff ligaments, tendons, and muscles, allowing you to move more freely.

Short, frequent stretches might help keep your muscles efficient throughout the day—this aids in maintaining appropriate posture and the reduction of aches and pains caused by tight muscles.

Supplementing senior-friendly strength training activities with a stretching regimen will assist in balancing out weaker muscles while also providing the benefits of flexibility to improve poor posture.

5. Stretching improves circulation and energy levels.

Stretching raises the temperature of your muscular tissue, resulting in increased circulation in that area. Circulation improves the health of your tissues.

Dynamic stretching is a low-intensity technique that involves moving your muscles in contrast to static stretching (stretching while your body is immobile).

Dynamic stretches help lengthen the muscles while increasing circulation and nutrition flow throughout your body. As a result, the body's energy levels rise. Increased energy is critical for preserving movement autonomy and maintaining social and healthy aging in older persons.

The following are some examples of dynamic stretches:

- Swinging arms
- Circles of the shoulders
- Lunges
- Swinging your legs
- Half squats

THE MUSCLES THAT NEED TO BE STRETCHED!

When practiced daily, these exercises can help you strengthen your flexibility:

Stretching the Hamstrings

This stretching exercise focuses on your lower back and legs, which is essential for senior flexibility. This stretch can help you stay mobile and fluid by reducing your leg and back stiffness.

To stretch the muscles at the back of the thigh, do the following:

- Sit on the floor with your legs in a V formation or straight ahead of you.
- Maintain a straight leg formation with toes pointed up.
- Lean forward slowly, take a deep breath and reach for your thigh, knee, or ankle.
- Hold the pose for 10-30 seconds if you feel a stretch at this point.

- Be careful not to hyperextend your hamstring when doing this stretch.
- If you don't feel a stretch in your leg on the bench, bend forward from your hips (not your waist).
- Keep your back and shoulders straight.
- Repeat with the opposite leg.
- Repeat 3-5 times on each side.

Standing Quadriceps Stretch

The standing quadriceps stretch is an excellent exercise for seniors since it is necessary for mobility and flexibility. The quadriceps muscle, which is located on the top part of your upper leg, is targeted in this exercise.

- Before stretching, make sure you limber yourself by performing some mild walking around.
- As you will be balancing on one leg for this exercise, grab a chair or the back of a couch for support. The greater the weight of the support, the better.
- With your left hand, hold on to the chair. Bend your right knee and grip your leg by the ankle with your right hand, gently pulling your foot towards your buttocks.
- Hold for 10 to 30 seconds before lowering your leg and repeating with your left leg.
- If you have trouble standing up, try the seated ankle stretch, which is also a helpful quadriceps stretch.

Stretching the Soleus

Another critical muscle group in your legs is the calf muscle, which will benefit from this simple stretch. The soleus stretch improves the deep calf muscle and the overall functionality of your legs, which helps your calves and lower body flexibility.

To stretch the lower leg muscles do the following:

- Stand with your arms outstretched and palms flat against the wall.

- Step back 1-2 feet (31-61 cm) with your right leg, heel, and foot flat on the floor, keeping your left knee bent slightly and the toes of your right foot slightly pointed inward.
- Your calf muscle should extend slightly but not to the point of discomfort. If you don't feel a stretch right away, move your foot back until you do.
- Maintain this position for 10 to 30 seconds.
- Bend your right leg's knee while keeping your heel and foot flat on the floor.
- Hold the position for 10 to 30 seconds more.
- Repeat with the other leg.
- Repeat this stretch exercise 3-5 times on each leg.

Ankle Stretch

To stretch muscles around the ankles, do the following:

- Take off your shoes.
- Sit towards the front edge of a chair and lean back, supporting your back with pillows.
- Your legs should be stretched out in front of you.
- Bend your ankles to point your feet toward you while keeping your heels on the floor.
- Point your feet away from you by bending your ankles.
- Repeat with your feet slightly off the floor if you don't feel the stretch.
- Hold the position for a few seconds.
- Repeat the same exercise on both feet 3 to 5 times.

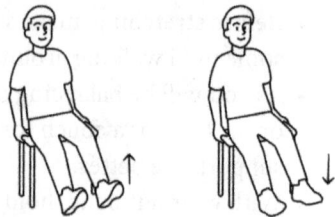

Rotation of a single hip

To stretch the pelvic and inner thigh muscles, do the following:

Note: If you've undergone a hip replacement, only undertake this exercise with your doctor's permission.

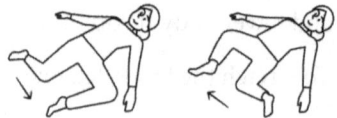

- Lie down on your back on the floor, knees bent, and feet flat on the ground.
- Keep your shoulders on the floor throughout the workout.
- Slowly lower one knee to the side while keeping the opposite leg and pelvis in position.
- Maintain this position for 10 to 30 seconds.
- Slowly return your knee to its original position.
- Repeat with the opposite knee.
- Repeat 3-5 times on each side.

Knee to Chest in a Seated Position

This lower body stretch is essential for seniors since it affects more than just their legs. The knee-to-chest stretching exercise increases hip and knee mobility by stretching the joints and improving lower back flexibility. This stretch has the extra benefit of not requiring you to stand.

To get started, follow these steps:

- Warm up your legs with gentle walking, similar to the previous workout.
- Sit comfortably in your chair and slowly draw your right knee towards your chest while seated.
- Hold this position for 10 to 30 seconds once you feel stretching.
- Return your leg to the floor gently and repeat the exercise with your other leg.

Advanced Standing Hip Flexor

This stretch is a terrific technique to relieve hip tightness or pain. However, it should be emphasized that it is a complicated exercise and is best suited for those with greater experience. This is how you do it:

- Take a chair and stand with your foot facing the chair's back, ensuring that you are far enough away from the chair to pull your leg up.
- Then, while holding both hands on the chair, keep one leg straight. Elevate your opposite leg towards your chest with your knee bent as close to your chest as possible.

- Hold this position for 10 to 15 seconds before switching to the other leg.

Stretching the Triceps

To stretch the muscles on the back of your upper arm, do the following:

- Hold one end of a towel in your right hand.
- Raise your right arm and bend it to drop the towel down your back.
- Continue to hold on to the towel with your right arm in this posture.
- With your left hand, reach behind your lower back and grab the bottom end of the towel.
- As you climb up the towel, your left hand will pull your right arm down.
- Continue until your hands are in contact or as close as you can get comfortable.
- Reverse the order of events.
- Each posture should be repeated 3-5 times.

The triceps stretch can be done while standing or sitting, just like the rest of our upper body exercises. Remember to keep your back straight by sitting tall and using a chair. Another easy way of stretching your triceps is given below.

- Place your feet hip-width apart and stand (or sit) tall.
- Raise both arms above your head, bending the right arm behind your head.
- Then, using your left hand on your right elbow, slowly draw your elbow down towards your back until you feel your upper arm stretching.
- Hold for 10 to 30 seconds, return your arms to their original positions, and repeat the stretch with your left arm.

Wrist Flexion

To stretch your wrist muscles, do the following:

- Place your hands in a praying position.

- Raise your elbows slowly until your arms are parallel to the floor and your hands are flat against each other.
- Stay in this position for 10-30 seconds.
- Repeat 3-5 times more.

Rotation of the Shoulders

To stretch the shoulder muscles, do the following:

- Lie down on the floor with a pillow under your head and your legs straight.
- Place a rolled towel between your knees if your back is bothering you.
- Straighten your arms out to the side.
- Keep your shoulders and upper arms flat on the floor throughout this exercise.
- Bend your elbows and point your hands towards the ceiling.
- Slowly roll your arms backward from the elbow. Stop when you feel a stretch or a tingling sensation, and immediately stop if you feel a pinching sensation or a sharp pain.
- Stay in this position for 10-30 seconds.
- Slowly raise your arms to point toward the ceiling, keeping your elbows bent. Then slowly roll your arms forward by bending your elbows to point toward your hips. When you feel a stretch or a slight discomfort, come to a halt.
- Maintain this position for 10 to 30 seconds
- Alternate between pointing over the head, toward the ceiling, and the hips.
- Begin and conclude with your finger pointed over your head.
- Repeat 3-5 times more.

Standing Side Stretch

The standing side stretch, also known as the overhead side stretch, is a practical and straightforward approach to loosening your tummy, back, and shoulders. To begin:

- Raise your arms over your head, interlocking your fingers, with your feet shoulder-width apart.

- Slowly lean to the left, keeping your torso long. Return to the center after holding this position for 10 to 30 seconds.
- Repeat the stretch on the right side.
- Another excellent feature of this workout is that it can be done while seated.
- This exercise can be done even with mobility or health issues.
- Keep your hips, knees, and toes looking forward while sitting in a tall chair if needed.
- Repeat the directions above with your arms raised over your head. (If this is too tough for you, put your arms on your hips or down by your sides.)
- Lean gently to one side for 10 to 30 seconds.

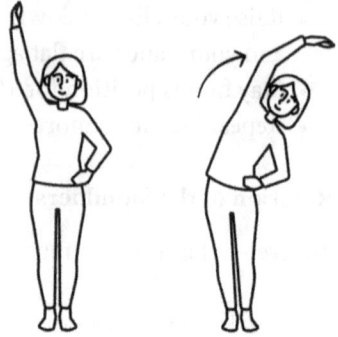

Neck Rotation

To stretch the neck muscles, do the following:

- Lie down on the floor with a phone book or other thick book propped up against your head.
- Turn your head slowly from side to side, keeping the position on each side for 10-30 seconds. Your head should not be tipped forward or backward; instead, it should be relaxed.
- To keep your back comfy, you can do this exercise with your knees bent.
- Repeat 3-5 times more.

Chair Lunge Stretch (Advanced)

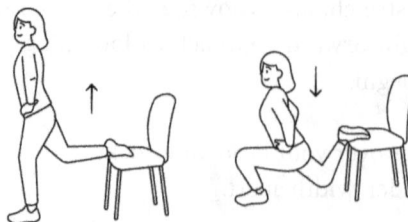

So far, we've discussed a few muscle groups and your upper and lower limbs, but what about the middle? This hip stretch is ideal for seniors who want to preserve their mobility and muscle strength.

To begin:

- Place two strong chairs approximately three feet apart and facing the same direction.
- Next, stand a few steps in front of the chair behind you and place your chin on the chair's seat. With your foot dangling over the back of the chair, your knee should extend just past the front border.
- Bend your front knee slightly while pushing your hips forward and down.
- Hold this position for 10 to 30 seconds before switching to the other side.

HOW MUCH AND HOW OFTEN YOU SHOULD STRETCH

The answer is daily if possible, but these are some suggestions from the National Institute on Aging:

- Combine flexibility exercises with endurance, strength, and balancing workouts to keep things new and exciting.
- Each stretch should be repeated 3-5 times.
- Slowly stretch each muscle group. Before relaxing, try to hold the stretch for 10-30 seconds. When repeating the stretch, strive to extend your arms further.

Safety Suggestions

- Consult your doctor before beginning a new workout routine.
- Be careful if you've had hip or knee replacement surgery.
- You must Warm-up your muscles before attempting to stretch them.
- Walking and moving your arms might assist your muscles in preparing for your workout.
- While a stretch may cause some discomfort, you should not be in pain. Stop stretching if you feel pain in any joint.

- Stretch slowly and gradually. Avoid bouncing or jerking, as these actions might cause harm.
- Avoid locking your joints while stretching. Maintain a slight bend in the limb instead.

When should you avoid stretching?

- Don't stretch when your range of motion is limited in some way; the flexibility movement can cause injury.
- There is inflammation or infection of the joint.
- A recent bone fracture or sprain has occurred in any part of the body.

What To Do After You've Stretched?

After you've finished your stretching exercises, you should think about other strategies to boost your health. Stretching exercises, proper hydration, and food all work together to assist seniors in maintaining their overall health. Stretching is just as crucial for elders as eating a balanced diet.

CHAPTER 3
STANDING STRONG
A GROUP OF STANDING EXERCISES

While elevating the foot during walking, we have to quickly shift our weight from one leg to the other to maintain the posture and balance of the body. We have to do the same while riding a bicycle. Standing on one leg for a few seconds, lifting our leg, and walking take strength, balance, and coordination.

But, as we age, it becomes more difficult to make rapid movements. Our coordination is lost with age. This imbalance often leads to severe falls in seniors. However, certain ways help us improve the balance and response rate of the body during rapid movements. Once you've practiced these exercises, your body will know what to do when you need to get your foot onto the ground quickly.

If you face these balance issues in older age, don't worry. In this chapter we will mention several exercises to help maintain your body's equilibrium. Incorporate these exercises into your daily life, and you will recognize the increase in your balance.

EXERCISE 1: TOE TAPS EXERCISE

Start with toe taps. Toe taps are a common exercise included in many training routines. Toe taps, like other fitness terminology, can refer to a variety of workouts that seem incredibly different from one another. Toe taps could refer to a movement you undertake as part of a pilates sequence (mind-body exercise) or an abdominal workout.

All of these toe taps have one thing in common: they all need the use of our core muscles to perform the movement.

Toe taps from a standing position

Standing toe taps are commonly used in warm-ups, conditioning drills for sports like soccer, between sets when lifting weights, and as part of a fitness class.

SCAN ME FOR VIDEO

This workout variation is excellent for:

- Increasing heart rate
- Targeting lower-body muscles
- Burning calories
- Improving speed, balance, and foot-handling skills

To perform a standing toe-tap correctly, you must have relatively strong glutes, hip flexors, quadriceps (front of thigh muscles), hamstrings (back of thigh), calves, and core muscles.

Depending on your chosen intensity, pumping your arms while tapping puts your upper body to work and raises the demands on your core muscles. Because the routine is cardio-based, you can expect your heart rate to rise and stay at a medium level throughout the workout.

Basic standing toe tap

This toe tap is suitable for people of all fitness levels. Items required for this exercise include a reading table, stair, wooden box, milk crate or any other stable structure 5 to 10 inches tall.

- Place yourself in front of a box, stair, crate or other stable surface.
- Place one foot on the platform's top.
- The ball of your foot will be in contact with the box or crate. Your other foot will stay on the ground, and your arms will be at your sides.
- First, push off with the planted foot, bringing it up and onto the stability platform while simultaneously lowering the lead foot to the floor. This transformation will occur in mid-flight.

- Land with the edge of the planted foot on the platform and the lead foot on the ground.
- Continue alternate feet for the required amount of time without pausing.
- The transition will be swift and feel like descending a flight of stairs.
- Do standing toe taps for 30 to 60 seconds.
- Repeat for 2 to 3 sets, resting for 15 to 30 seconds between sets.
- Increase the tempo of the toe taps and pump your arms to make this technique more difficult if it doesn't hurt you.

To alleviate the difficulty, you can execute toe taps on the ground, using the identical movements as above but without the higher step.

Try one of these variations if you want to change how you make the move

Modified Toe Tap

You can alter the maneuver and still have excellent outcomes. The hop and landing are removed from this version of the exercise.

- Keep both feet on the ground in front of a box or other stable platform
- Begin by elevating and tapping your right foot on the platform
- Then, repeat this with your left foot while your right foot is on the floor
- Alter sides, but don't switch mid-flight
- During the transition, both feet should be in contact with the ground
- Alternate feet for the specified amount of time
- Do standing toe taps for 30 to 60 seconds
- Repeat the same for 2 to 3 sets

Benefits of Toe Taps

- The muscles targeted by toe taps are the quadriceps, hamstrings, glutes, hip flexors, and calves.
- They also help strengthen your core, resulting in less back pain, excellent balance, and increased trunk flexion, extension, and rotation.

- You're also working your cardiovascular system by repeatedly tapping each foot.
- Adding toe taps to your existing workout will help you raise your heart rate and burn more calories while strengthening your muscles.
- The movement pattern in toe-tap exercise helps your body prepare for more advanced activities like leaping lunges and plyometric box jumps.
- They may even help you enhance your jump height and walking speed.

Regularly performing toe taps as a functional strength exercise can make it simpler to complete everyday activities that require similar movements, such as climbing the stairs.

EXERCISE 2: SQUATS

A squat is one of the most effective leg-strengthening exercises. It engages all of the leg muscles as well as the core. It's also a movement you do throughout the day, such as lifting items or standing in particular positions. Remember, we never bend down to pick up or move something heavy from behind. We rely on stronger muscles, such as our legs and glutes (buttocks).

SCAN ME FOR VIDEO

Perfect your squat technique to engage the muscles and avoid excessive strain efficiently. So, without further ado, here's how you properly squat. (Why don't you get up right now and practice it - it's a crucial exercise that will tremendously assist you).

How to Squat?

- Standing tall with your feet shoulder-width apart is an excellent start.
- The toes might point forward or slightly outwards.
- Hold on to your chair with both hands, or keep your arms straight out in front for balance.
- Engage your core, bend at the hips, then sit back as if sitting in a chair.

- Maintain a 90-degree angle as you sit back, keeping your chest high and your core firm.
- As you stand back up, distribute your weight evenly between both legs, keeping your heels on the floor.
- Ensure your knees stay in line with your toes throughout the exercise; they should not move past your toes or inward.

Why the squat is such a beneficial workout for seniors and the elderly

The squat is a beneficial exercise for people of all ages. It's a wonderful exercise for elderly folks to help maintain an evenly developed muscle mass in their legs.

- During the squat, all the lower body muscles are engaged (including the core).
- Not only that, but the squat perfectly replicates the movement patterns of standing to sitting and sitting to standing. Consider how many times you sit and stand throughout the day. Quite a few times!
- As you get older, improving your strength in one particular movement pattern can significantly impact your quality of life and independence.

How many squats should you do as a senior?

Our bodies can adapt to a wide range of situations. Our muscles (including the heart) will not become stronger if we do not put any stress on them. Indeed, the aging process weakens our muscles over time.

When you undertake resistance workouts regularly, your body learns to adapt and get stronger. Because we can feel it, the amount of tension you put on your muscles is pretty easy to determine.

If you try to complete 100 squats, you'll most likely feel exhausted and experience pain in your legs long before reaching that number. Doing as many squats as comfortably possible until you feel fatigued would be best. Fatigue is a sign that you're putting strain on your muscles, which means they'll adapt, grow, and become stronger.

Will bodyweight squats suffice to increase strength?

Yes, most certainly, at first. But don't forget the adaptability of your body. After exercising bodyweight squats daily, your body will adapt to the stress level and settle.

You can increase your stress levels in a variety of ways.

- Increase the number of reps or sets.
- Hold a lightweight during the exercise.
- The tempo of activity can be slowed or sped up.

These are all excellent examples of increasing stress. Progressive overload is a more popular term for it. Some individuals carry water bottles as a weight, while others carry a few books in their backpacks.

Home workouts may be beneficial in increasing strength and mobility as an older person with a bit of imagination.

Muscles involved in Squats

The squat is an example of a compound movement, which simultaneously engages two or more muscles. The quadriceps, glutes, and hamstrings are the key muscles used in the squat, and these three muscles comprise a significant amount of the lower body's musculature. You'll have more mobility and confidence if all three muscle groups are strong.

Are squats bad for older individuals?

You might think that squats are bad for seniors, but the answer is entirely different. Squats are not harmful to the elderly. They are often quite good for older individuals to do. Squats imitate the most typical movement pattern we do daily. Claiming that squats are harmful is like saying that standing and sitting are both terrible. It's completely absurd!

Squats can be difficult, especially if you suffer from arthritis. It's permissible, though, to employ adjustments and tools to help you squat. Using the arms or the back of a chair are excellent ways to simplify squats. When you exercise, it's natural to have some pain in an arthritic joint. Adapt the movement to reduce any discomfort you may be experiencing.

EXERCISE 3: SINGLE-LEG STANCE EXERCISE

Single leg exercises help regain balance and increase the strength of your lower body. Here is how you can do this exercise at home.

- Stand next to a chair for safety and stability.
- Stand on one leg.
- Hold this position for as long as feasible for you, and keep note of your time if necessary.
- Alternate your feet once you've completed the assigned time.
- If you're having trouble with this exercise, you can use two seats, one on each side of you.
- Close your eyes and practice holding for the stated period to make this exercise more challenging.
- This exercise can also be done on an unstable surface, such as a cushion.
- Alternatively, you might include a task, such as bouncing a ball.

EXERCISE 4: TANDEM STANCE EXERCISE

Here is how to perform a tandem stance exercise.

- In a "heel-toe" stance, stand with one foot in front of the other.
- If this is too tough at first, spread your feet slightly apart. As needed, use a counter or chair for support.
- Hold this position for 10 seconds on each side.
- Repeat it 2–3 times more.

Why this exercise is significant

This practice is beneficial because it forces you to have a restricted perspective. Your muscles will work harder to keep you balanced with a smaller support base.

EXERCISE 5: WEIGHT SHIFTING EXERCISES

A balanced exercise program for seniors must include weight-shifting exercises to teach them about their center of gravity to enhance balance and prevent falls. Weight-shifting exercises can help with coordination, lower-extremity muscle strength, and slower, more accurate motions.

SCAN ME FOR VIDEO

For active older individuals, here are some weight-shifting exercises to try:

NORMAL WEIGHT SHIFTING EXERCISE

- Stand with your feet hip-width apart
- Shift your body weight on the right foot.
- Raise your left foot off the ground.
- Hold this position for up to 30 seconds.
- Then repeat on the other side.
- Repeat the same on each leg three times.

Side Sways

- Place your feet slightly wider than hip-width apart while seated or standing.
- Lean the body somewhat to the right, leading with the upper body while keeping both feet on the floor.
- Repeat in the opposite direction.
- Rep 10–15 times more.

EXERCISE 6: ALTERNATE LEG IN AND OUT EXERCISE

Here is how you can do an alternate leg in and out exercise.

- Place yourself in front of a counter.
- Hold on with both hands.
- Lift one leg out to the side, with toes pointing to the front.
- Hold for a few seconds before slowly lowering the leg.
- Repeat with the other leg.
- Continue until you've completed 3–4 times on each side.
- Increase the number of reps until you can accomplish 15 on each leg.
- Reduce the amount of assistance you give with your hands over time.

EXERCISE 7: SHORT LUNGES FOR SENIORS

Follow the following steps to perform short lunges.

SCAN ME FOR VIDEO

- Stand with your arms by your sides and your feet hip-width apart.
- Keep your chin, shoulder blades, and core sturdy and aligned.
- Inhale deeply, take a step forward, and lower your body to the floor by bending your front legs knee and hip by 30 degrees.
- Exhale and return to a standing position by squeezing your buttocks.
- Repeat.

Benefits of Lunges for Seniors

Lunges are an excellent exercise for seniors and older adults for various reasons. The lunge, like the squat, is a compound activity, which means it works for two or more main muscle groups simultaneously. The quads, glutes, and hamstrings are all engaged during the lunge.

Most of the strain will be in the quads if the torso is kept more upright during the exercise (front of the upper leg). The tension is moved more onto the glutes and hamstrings if the torso swings forward more throughout the exercise (back of the upper leg)

Because you are just training one limb at a time, the lunge is also a unilateral activity. A unilateral movement can be pretty beneficial in balancing muscular imbalances between the limbs.

The most common mistakes that older people make while performing lunges

One of the most common mistakes is when the front foot's heel comes off the ground during the lunge movement. The front foot should remain flat throughout the movement. The front leg should be responsible for around 80% or more of the weight distribution. The back leg serves primarily as support. Keeping the feet hip-width apart during the exercise is also a good idea. There will be a lot more balance as a result of this.

Another difficulty is people's failure to grasp a sturdy object for help. It's quite acceptable to do so and is encouraged. Having a light hold of an item, such as a chair, can aid balance, allowing you to focus on pushing through that front leg.

How many reps and sets of lunges should I do as an older adult?

Various factors will determine the number of lunge reps you execute. You need to know that there are a few "must-do" things for your body to adapt and become stronger. The cornerstones of an effective strength-building program are the three items listed below.

- How many sets and reps do you do per week?
- How many times each week do you exercise?
- Intensity, it refers to how hard you push yourself during each set and workout.

Programming is the process of combining these three elements with the right exercises. For progress to be made, effective programming is required. It's pointless to add a few lunges to your regimen on the spur of the moment.

EXERCISE 8: HEEL RAISE EXERCISE

- Standing with your feet shoulder-width apart is the best way to start.
- Lift your heels off the ground while holding onto a counter or a hard surface.
- You should feel most of your weight move to the front of your feet as if you're standing on your toes.
- It's OK to put your palms onto the counter first; ensure you're standing erect and not slouching.
- Reduce the pressure you apply with your arms and eventually let go of the counter to progress this workout.
- Make a few repetitions of the same process.

SCAN ME FOR VIDEO

Muscles Involved in Heel Raise Exercise

· The gastrocnemius and soleus muscles, located in the calf area, are worked by the heel raise.

Significance

The heel raise, often known as the heel lift, provides a variety of advantages. Your calf muscle aids with balance as it governs the position of your ankle. You'll use your ankle muscles to adjust when you're shaky or need to correct your balance. Better balance comes from stronger calf muscles. You will regain the spring in your step by doing the entire heel raise exercise. You might even have the opportunity to try out some new dance skills.

Sitting Heel Raise

- Take a seat in a chair.
- Your feet should be 6 to 8 inches apart, level on the floor, and parallel to one another.
- Raise your heels to get on the balls of your feet.
- Return to the starting position and repeat the motion 10 to 15 times more.
- Complete at least two sets of 10 to 15 repetitions.

Standing Heel Raise with the help of a Chair

- Stand in front of a chair with your face towards the back.
- Feet should be 6 to 8 inches apart, level on the ground, and parallel to one another.
- Make a slight bend in your knees to avoid locking them.
- Raise your heels off the ground and onto the balls of your feet.
- Use the back of the chair for balance when moving.
- Return to the starting position and repeat the motion 10 to 15 times more.
- Complete at least two sets of 10 to 15 repetitions.

Things to consider while performing Heel Raises

Because the range of motion involved in a heel raise is limited, be careful to do heel raise exercises to the fullest extent possible. Also, strive to keep a steady speed throughout your repetitions. There will be no bouncing or jerking up and down.

EXERCISE 9: MARCHING IN PLACE EXERCISE

Marching in place is a low-impact exercise that helps people lose weight. Marching in place is a fantastic way for those who are overweight or obese to gain cardio without the risk of injury that comes with high-impact exercise. Marching in place is an excellent starting point for individuals new to fitness. The development levels for this activity come effortlessly.

Try introducing arm movements, up and down overhead, as you march to integrate full-body training once you've mastered marching in place. Once you gain confidence, you can raise the intensity of your march and turn it into a light jog in place. Remember to listen to your body; we all have various fitness degrees and different amounts of activities that challenge us.

EXERCISE 10: SHOULDER ROLLS

Shoulder Rolls are one of the most common shoulder exercises. This exercise strengthens the shoulder blades to allow for more vigorous lifting and increases shoulder mobility when shrugging. Here is how you can do this exercise perfectly.

SCAN ME FOR VIDEO

- Sit or stand with your feet shoulder-width apart and weights in your hands. Then, raise the shoulders toward the ears. If you do not have weights that is fine as well, some people use makeshift weights such as bottles of water or heavier household items. Then, raise the shoulders toward the ears.
- Bring the shoulders down and backward.
- Make 20 repetitions.
- Exhale as your shoulders rise and fall.
- Lift the rib cage, flex the knees slightly, and tuck the chin inwards.
- Only move from the shoulders, which should go as high as possible.
- Keep the elbows fully extended.

EXERCISE 11: WALL PUSHUPS

Push-ups are an excellent workout for strengthening the upper body muscles. Still, they are too tough for most people to complete correctly. A proper way of doing wall push-ups for seniors is to:

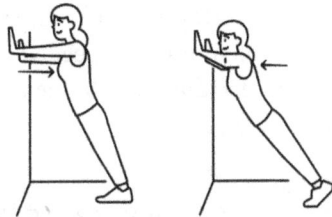

- Stand approximately an arm's length away from the wall, facing it.
- Place your hands on the wall with your fingers pointing up.
- Your hands should be below shoulder level and broader than shoulder-width apart.
- Bend your elbows and bring your head between your hands to the wall.
- Your entire body should pivot at the ankles and move forward.
- There should be no movement of the feet.
- Then push your body away from the wall to return to your starting position.

Gravity pushes down your entire body as you try to push yourself up, making a standard push-up quite tricky. We considerably lessen the influence of gravity on the movement by performing this exercise in this position.

Push-ups on the counter (Advanced)

This is a variation of the same exercise. The edge of a countertop is used instead of the wall.

- You'll have to shift your feet backward a little after placing your hands on the countertop, which should be slightly broader than shoulder-width apart.
- Then bend your elbows, lower your chest to the countertop, and press back up to the starting position.
- Maintain a straight line from your ankles to your shoulders by keeping your body in a straight line.

You'll note that this is more difficult than the wall version. Gravity exerts additional resistance since you are leaning forward at a greater angle. Both exercises' difficulty is primarily determined by how deep down you go. It will be far more challenging to lower your head or chest to the wall or countertop than to simply drop it merely a few inches. Adjust your range of motion as needed. You can test both variants of the Push-up before deciding which one is ideal for you. Do this exercise 10 times, 2-3 times a week.

EXERCISE 12: STANCE EXERCISES FOR BALANCE

Normal stance

Your feet should be around hip distance apart in a typical posture. This indicates that your feet are directly beneath your hip bones. When someone says, "stand with your feet hip-width apart."

If you ask most people to stand normally, they will choose this stance, which is also the position from which most of us begin walking.

Narrow Stance

- The feet are placed close together in a narrow stance.

- Begin by putting your feet together or as near as you can while remaining steady.
- Stand tall and stretch forward with one hand while holding onto a counter or other surface to keep yourself safe.
- As you stretch ahead, switch arms.
- Reaching forward with both hands is an excellent way to start. Reaching out to the side or in different directions can be more difficult.
- Make ten reaches with each arm. Repeat it for 2–3 times.

Why is a narrow stance significant?

Many older people fall while reaching for something in a confined place. This practice helps you maintain your equilibrium in such situations.

Lower Center of Gravity

The center of gravity for most people is a place in the belly just below the navel. It is somewhat in front of the spine.

- Put a tiny bend in your knees from your wider stance, which will lower your center of gravity by a few inches.
- This should feel even more steady because the modest knee bend encourages you to activate the muscles in your midsection, hips, and legs and lower your center of gravity.

EXERCISE 13: THREE-WAY HIP KICK

Hip discomfort, knee pain, and even foot pain (such as plantar fasciitis or posterior tibialis syndrome) can be accompanied by external hip rotation deficits. The deep hip superficial rotator muscles must act in unison with other hip external rotators and hip abductors to ensure correct lower extremity alignment when the leg is fully weight-bearing.

The leg takes complete weight-bearing during walking, jogging, skipping, or landing from a leap while the opposite leg

is in the swing phase.

Here is how you can do a three-way hip kick exercise.

- Stand with your feet shoulder-width.
- Extend your leg forward and return to your starting position while holding onto a counter or sturdy surface.
- Repeat the move to the side, returning to the initial position each time.
- Finally, return to the beginning position by extending your leg back.
- On each leg, repeat each action 5 to 10 times.
- Repeat the complete steps 2–3 times.

Significance

This exercise strengthens the hip muscles, providing stability when walking, turning, climbing, and descending stairs.

The standing hip 3-way exercise is a simple and efficient approach to strengthening leg muscles. The key to this exercise is to:

- Keep the stance knee unlocked and in a "soft" stance with the patella (knee cap) rotated slightly outside (laterally) (usually pointing toward the 3rd or 4th toe).
- The hip, not the ankle, must be used to rotate.
- The primary focus should be on hip stability and activation of the deep hip external rotators.

EXERCISE 14: SIDE STEPPING

- Start standing with your feet together.
- Step to the side, keeping your hands on a counter or a sturdy surface until your feet are just past shoulder width.
- Move along a counter, 5 to 10 steps on each side.
- Repeat 2–3 times more.

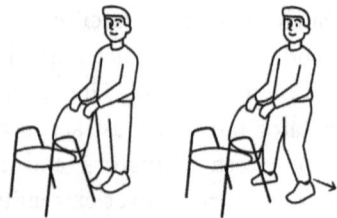

Importance of Side Stepping

Many older persons fall because of poor coordination when turning and stepping in confined places. This practice will help you improve your coordination for all the rotations and side-steps you'll do throughout the day.

Imagine yourself standing on one foot (but don't try it unless you have something to grip onto). Your support base on one foot is only 4 or 5 inches wide, and a light breeze might easily knock you over. And when you take a step, what do you do? You balance for a split second on one foot while bringing the other to the front. It's critical to keep your capacity to balance on a minimal support base as you get older if you want to keep your mobility and freedom.

Conclusion

All the standing exercises can help you improve the coordination of the body while also enhancing the strength of muscles and balance, preventing falls. Always contact your doctor before starting a new workout routine and check for any pain or other side effects. Start every exercise slowly, and then stretch that to your bearable limit.

CHAPTER 4
SITTING IN STRENGTH
A GROUP OF SEATED EXERCISES

Most seniors face difficulty moving around independently and find it difficult to get even a small amount of exercise throughout the day. In that case, they shouldn't worry too much because there are still ways to exercise without even going to the gym.

Seated chair exercises are an excellent option if you face mobility and balance issues in old age.

Remember that there is no requirement for a weight set or a trainer, and you do not need to be accompanied by a caregiver. The main thing you need is a chair; however, some of the following exercises may require a resistance band or dumbbells for optimal results.

THE BENEFITS OF SEATED EXERCISES

Although not everyone in old age can move quickly or even get out of their chair, this should not prevent them from exercising. While using a chair as mobility equipment, you can conduct various normal activities. The chair should be stable with no wheels or rollers.

In this chapter we will discuss the seated exercises for seniors in detail to help you visualize how to perform each exercise correctly. Complete each exercise according to the specified time, repetitions, and sets.

EXERCISE 15: SIT TO STAND EXERCISES

Being able to stand up from a chair significantly impacts the daily lives of seniors. It assists with basic tasks such as getting up from the toilet, getting out of bed, and getting out of a chair. As a result, the sit-to-stand exercise is one of the finest mobility exercises.

It's a functional workout that improves leg, core, and back muscles for that specific movement. These muscles are required to improve mobility, independence, and balance.

SCAN ME FOR VIDEO

Unlike other exercises, sit-to-stand exercise does not require any special equipment and can be done anywhere if you have a chair. Here is an overview of the exercise instructions and suggestions for how many repetitions to perform and how to keep your elderly relative safe while exercising.

- Take a seat in a chair that has a solid surface. A solid surface is recommended because a soft chair or couch makes it harder for seniors to stand up.
- Lean your body forward until your nose and toes are in line.
- Use your legs to push yourself up to get out of the chair. Try not to use your hands to assist you in getting out of the chair.
- Once standing erect, squeeze your glutes to extend your hips fully.
- Hold this position for one second, then slowly lower yourself back into the chair without plopping down.
- Repeat ten times more.
- Rest for a minute, then repeat for three sets of ten reps.
- To make this practice a little more challenging, follow these instructions:
- Place yourself in front of a chair.
- Slowly lower yourself toward the chair by pushing your hips back. Make sure you're leaning backward and your knees aren't crossing your toes.
- lightly tap the chair with your buttocks, then stand up.
- Repeat ten times more.

- Rest for a minute, then repeat for three sets of ten reps.

EXERCISE 16: KNEE EXTENSION EXERCISES

Maintaining your functional independence requires standing fully and effortlessly, extending your knee. The joints lose part of their flexibility and range of motion as we age. Seniors should do knee strengthening exercises to keep their balance and avoid falling. The knee extension exercise listed below is the easiest knee rehab exercise. Ensure your knee is fully extended and flexed to get the most out of this exercise.

- Sit in a chair as comfortably as possible, with your hips as far back as feasible.
- Make sure your back is firmly attached to the chair's backrest.
- Maintain a tight core and extend your chest.
- Place your hands at the sides of the chair and grab the seat to stay stable.
- Maintain a 90-degree angle with the chair with both legs.
- Extend one leg in front of the body until it is fully extended in the air.
- Keep the opposite leg in its original posture for stability.
- Before lowering your leg back down, hold for a few seconds. At the apex of the action, squeeze the muscles at the front of your thigh.
- Make sure you're moving slowly and steadily.
- Slowly return one leg to its original position.
- Alter your legs, ensuring that your knees are fully extended (leg completely straight).
- To count as one set, repeat for both legs.

EXERCISE 17: HEEL SLIDES

Heel slides are simple leg workouts in which you have to extend your leg away from your body, bend your knee, and then slide your heel toward your buttocks. These exercises can be done on a bed, the floor, or the wall and are frequently advised after a knee injury or hip surgery.

Heel slides are used to expand the range of motion in your knee and strengthen the tissues to improve stability. Depending on your needs, you can perform one or more types of heel slides. Each type of heel slide works on a different set of muscles.

When practicing this exercise, keep the following points in mind:

- Slide your heel as close as possible to your buttocks.
- Bend your knee to a comfortable extent.
- You may feel pressure around your knee, but it shouldn't hurt.
- Perform 1 to 3 sets of 10 repetitions for each exercise.
- Take a minute to rest between the sets.
- Perform these exercises at least twice a day.

Normal Heel Slides

You can play about with the position of your toes. Draw your toes towards the shin. Alternatively, you can turn your toes to either side. Follow these instructions to perform regular heel slides.

- Sit-down on the ground, extend your legs and put your feet slightly apart.
- Place a towel around one foot, and hold the towel with both hands.
- Now slide the towel leg as close to your buttocks as possible, using the towel as an aid.
- Stay in this position for a total of 5 seconds.
- Return your heel to the beginning position by sliding it backward.

Heel slides for abduction and adduction

During this exercise, maintain hip and leg alignment by pointing your knee and foot toward the ceiling.

- Lie down on your back, extend your legs and keep your feet slightly apart.
- Point your toes or simply draw them towards your shin.
- Now slowly slide one leg out to the side.

- Return your leg to the starting position without bringing it past your body's midline.

Seated Heel Slides

- To perform this exercise, you must sit in a chair and extend your leg.
- Slide your heel back to the chair as much as possible.
- Hold the position for 5 seconds.
- Return your foot to the initial position by sliding it backward.
- Repeat the same on the other leg

Things to Consider Before Heel Slides Exercise

- Start with a warm-up for at least 5 minutes before beginning these workouts.
- Try using a heating pad on your knee for a few minutes if you can't get up and walk or move about.
- Keep in mind that your body may feel less flexible in the morning.
- Massage your knee before and after doing heel slides.
- Use essential oils blended with a carrier oil, a CBD topical, or a muscle rub for the best results.
- Placing a plastic bag under your heel makes it easier to slide on a carpet or a bed.
- If you are working out on a hard floor, you can wear socks or lay a towel beneath your heels.
- Slow, deliberate movements are recommended. Avoid jerky, rapid movements.
- Press your low back to the floor or place a folded towel under it for support.
- Avoid raising your neck by using your core muscles.
- You can also wrap a strap or towel around your foot to move easier.

Muscles Involved in this Exercise

Heel slides improve quadriceps, hamstrings, and calf strength. They also strengthen the muscles and tissues that surround the knee. Heel slides help prevent and treat low back pain by strengthening the core muscles, aiding general body stability, and beneficial to all motions.

Benefits of Heel Slides

Heel slides are commonly used to help people recover from surgery or injuries. They are a simple way to keep your body active if you cannot move around freely. Heel slides improve mobility, flexion, and flexibility by increasing the range of motion in your knee.

They also aid in strengthening the muscles, ligaments, and tendons in your hips and legs. Furthermore, using heel slides to keep your leg active lowers discomfort and improves circulation, allowing you to feel better overall.

They may also be beneficial in treating Baker's cysts and fibromyalgia flare-ups and symptoms.

Caution

While you may experience some sensation or discomfort during these exercises, you should immediately stop if you experience any pain. When initially starting, go softly and gently with your movements.

Make sure you're at ease throughout the process. If you press yourself into a position, your knee will be put under stress. If you can only bend your knee slightly, that's fine. Gradually, you'll be able to bend your knee fully.

Ice your knee for 20 minutes if it feels uncomfortable after the workouts or during the day. This can aid in the reduction of discomfort. Ice your knee multiple times every day. Rest and elevate your leg as much as possible for the most significant outcomes.

Final Words About Heel Slides

Heel slides can be done independently or as part of a more extensive training routine. Increase your strength and stability while increasing your mobility and range of motion. Experiment and pick the most beneficial versions of heel slides for your body.

See a fitness or healthcare professional if you're not sure which exercises are good for you. Listen to your body, and don't overwork yourself, especially if you're recovering from surgery or an injury. Continue to do these exercises regularly as you recuperate and progress to retain your results.

EXERCISE 18: SEATED CALF RAISES

The calf raise may assist in stretching stiff muscles or joints in the lower half of the leg if a senior has trouble squatting.

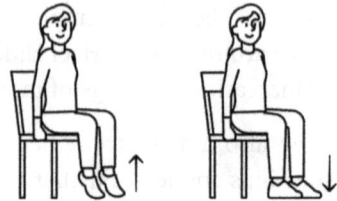

Steps:

- Sit in the chair with your hips as far back as feasible.
- Make sure your back is firmly attached to the chair's backrest.
- Maintain a tight core (abdominals and lumbar spine). Extend your chest.
- To stay stable, place both hands at the sides of the chair and grab the seat.
- Maintain a 90-degree angle with the chair with both legs. Place both feet flat on the ground.
- Extend the heels of your feet slowly upward, keeping your toes on the ground and your heels in the air.
- Return both feet to their original positions.
- Repeat this action for 20 reps or more.
- Place a medicine ball or similar weight of equivalent value near the edge of the lap if this activity feels too simple with simply bodyweight (almost to the knees).
- Alternatively, place a shallow object beneath both feet (approximately 3-4 inches off the ground) for a full range of motion.

Muscles Used in Calf Raise:

The soleus and gastrocnemius muscles are two different muscles in your calves. Though it's difficult to see, the soleus muscle traverses the length of your lower leg and aids in movement. The gastrocnemius connects the knee to the top of the calves. The soleus is primarily targeted with sitting raises. A standing calf raise increases the attention on the gastrocnemius.

Who can do This Exercise?

This workout is suitable for anyone free of a lower-body injury.

How Many Calf Raises Should You Do While Sitting?

If you're new to exercise, start by completing three sets of 10 to 12 repetitions. Calves are prone to delayed muscular discomfort, so get a sense of how your body reacts before increasing the stress.

Benefits of Calf Raise Exercise

The calf raises exercise's main advantage is increased muscle strength and growth. While this alters the appearance of your legs, it also increases their performance. Your entire leg will work better if your calves are more muscular. This exercise can also help avoid ankle injuries because the soleus hooks into your ankle. It can also help you prevent injuries to your shins and knees.

EXERCISE 19: SEATED MARCHING

This exercise strengthens the hip flexor muscles responsible for pulling the leg up, crucial for walking and climbing stairs. Hip flexor weakness can make walking difficult by decreasing the length of your steps and slowing down your walking speed. Increased difficulty lifting the legs when walking reduces foot clearance, which increases the danger of foot drag, leading to trips and falls. Follow the steps below to perform this exercise:

SCAN ME FOR VIDEO

- Sit in a chair with your arms at your sides and your back straight.
- Begin by marching with your legs alternating. Return to the beginning position by raising one thigh as high as possible, then repeat with the other leg.
- Pump your arms if you can.
- Continue for another 30 seconds, or perform a total of 20 marches.

EXERCISE 20: SEATED TOE TAPS

This toe-tapping exercise can assist with developing core muscles. Core strengthening exercises (stomach and back) can aid with weight balance, mobility, the prevention and reduction of chronic back and neck discomfort. Here is how you can perform seated toe taps:

- Sit on a chair with your legs out in front of you. Keep your toes pointing upwards without bending your knees.
- Place both hands on your thighs and sit erect by keeping your head aligned with your spine.
- Now you have to tighten your abdominal muscles to stabilize the spine.
- Softly exhale and bend forward from your hips, moving your hands down your legs towards your ankles.
- Keep your back flat by avoiding rounding your back towards the ceiling.
- Maintain a neutral spine alignment with your head, legs extended, and toes pointed upwards towards the ceiling.
- Continue to bend and extend forward until the stretch reaches a point of tension.
- Avoid pushing yourself to the point of discomfort.
- Hold this position for 15 to 30 seconds, then return to your starting position and repeat 2-4 times.
- You can choose to hold this position by grasping your ankles.

EXERCISE VARIATION:

To make this stretch more dynamic, conduct slow, controlled motions for 1 set of 5 to 10 repetitions, holding the stretched posture for 1 to 2 seconds each time.

Stretch simply to the point of tension, avoiding bouncing, and controlling movement at other parts of the body are critical ways to optimize the benefits of a stretch while reducing the risk of damage. Avoid rounding your low back too much during this exercise.

EXERCISE 21: SEATED ARM RAISES

The overhead arm raise is a good workout for strengthening the muscles in your upper limbs. You need a pair of lightweights or two water bottles and a solid, preferably armless chair for this exercise.

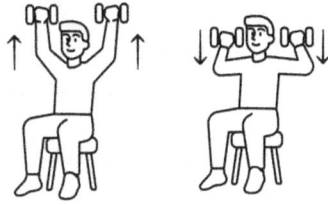

- Put your feet flat on the floor and sit tall.
- Begin by gripping a weight in each hand, bending your elbows, and holding the weights to the sides of your shoulders and palms facing forward.
- Repeat by pressing the weights above your head, holding for a count of one, and then lowering the weights to the beginning position.
- Do 10 to 12 repetitions in each set, then rest for a minute before repeating.

An alternate way to strengthen your arms and shoulders by doing seated arm raises is given below. Choose the method which seems more comfortable for you.

- Sit in your chair with your feet shoulder-width apart on the ground.
- Raise both arms straight in front of you, palms facing you.
- Now raise both arms above your head simultaneously.
- Return your arms to their elevated posture.
- Next, spread each arm, one to the left and the other to the right of your body, making the letter T.
- Return your arms to their original elevated position.
- This is one rep; repeat ten times for three reps.
- Take a minute to rest between sets.

Focusing on Biceps in Arm Raises

Arm curls are a great way to strengthen the muscles at the front of your upper arm. Here is how you can do this exercise.

Hold a weight in each hand while sitting in your chair. Let your arms hang by the sides of the chair.

- Begin with your palms facing inward.
- Bend your right elbow and increase the weight to the front of your shoulder.
- Turn your hand so that your palm faces up halfway through the action.
- Lower the weight to the beginning position after a one-count pause.
- To finish one repetition, repeat with your left hand.
- Alternate arms until you've completed 10 to 12 repetitions.
- Perform a second set after a minute of rest.

Strengthening Triceps with Arm Raises

This exercise focuses on strengthening the muscles on the back of your arm.

- Use only one hand weight and triceps extensions to develop the muscles in the rear of your upper arm.
- Sit in a chair and place your feet flat on the floor.
- Now lean forward slightly, and place your right forearm across both legs to support your upper body.
- Turn your left hand so your palm faces the body and holds the weight in your left hand.
- Bend your elbow 90 degrees and move your arm backward until your upper arm is parallel to the floor while maintaining this angle.

This is where you'll begin.

- Straighten your left arm to the extent that it becomes parallel to the floor without moving your upper arm.
- Rep 10 to 12 times more from the beginning position.
- Repeat with your right hand as the weight.

THINGS TO CONSIDER IN ARM STRENGTHENING EXERCISES

Start with either 1lb or 2 lb hand weights, depending on your strength level, and progressively raise the weight as you gain strength. If you don't have hand weights, two soup cans or two water bottles can be substituted. Just make sure they suit your hand and are comfortable to grasp..

EXERCISE 22: BACK EXTENSION WITH AN ISOMETRIC HAND

The back extension hold is a simple isometric back extension strength and endurance exercise.

Execution

Here is the easiest guide to doing this exercise.

SCAN ME FOR VIDEO

- Sit up straight in your chair.
- Squeeze your shoulder blades to create strength and stiffness in your muscles.
- Keep your core tight and your arms to the side parallel to the ground.
- Hinge forward and hold for a moment.
- One rep is bringing yourself back up.
- Repeat the same steps for two sets of 10 repetitions each.

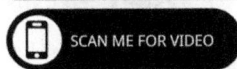

Purpose

The back extension hold is a simple approach to increase back extensor stamina, which can aid in maintaining desirable posture in other exercises or build the capacity to maintain that back arch when loaded with greater resistance. The activity can be performed unweighted for brief periods of moderate effort as part of a warm-up to prepare the trunk or for more extended periods and with added resistance at the end of training sessions. Three to Four sets of 1 to 3 days per week is sufficient.

Variations

Depending on the personal needs, the back extension hold can be performed with a complete arch or a position closer to a neutral spine position.

EXERCISE 23: SEATED TORSO TWISTS

The sitting torso twist strengthens the core, particularly the obliques, and improves spinal mobility. Here is how you can do seated torso twists.

SCAN ME FOR VIDEO

- Sit tall with your feet about hip-distance apart on the ground.
- Make sure you're not slouching in your chair.
- Keep your hands behind your head, elbows bent, and pointed out to the sides of the room.
- Exhale and then slowly twist your body to the right side comfortably while keeping your pelvis stable.
- Return to the center on an inhale, keeping your hips stable.
- Take a deep exhale and rotate your torso to the left as comfortably as possible.
- Return to the center with an inhale.
- Continue until you've twisted six to eight times on each side.
- Perform a second set after a brief rest.

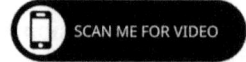

FINAL WORDS

Muscle strength can improve balance and stability, lowering the chance of falling. It's also easier to get through the day when you're stronger. Life becomes more enjoyable when you can travel around with ease. Lifting heavy bags and other items that once weighed you down can remind you of your improved fitness and health.

If mobility limitations prevent you from completing seated or standing workouts, there are modifications you can make to get the same benefits. A good suggestion is doing the exercise with a limited range of motion. Don't lift your arms aloft with the dumbbell overhead press if you have pain, shoulder mobility issues, or both. Instead, go only three-quarters or halfway up or as high as you're comfortable with.

It's natural to experience mobility limitations as you get older, primarily due to poor posture and prolonged sitting over the years. Listen to your body and combine your workouts with a flexibility and mobility routine.

Physical fitness is essential for everyone, and our needs may alter as we age. Exercise programs that accommodate limited mobility can help you stay active while improving strength and range of motion.

If you are finding this book useful, please take 60 seconds to leave a review so others can take advantage of these cool concepts, as reviews help others find what they need. Thank you so much for your attention and participation!
https://www.amazon.com/review/create-review?&asin=B0C2B2JQ9P

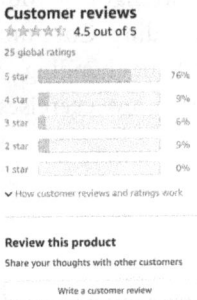

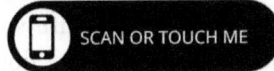

Customer reviews
★★★★½ 4.5 out of 5
25 global ratings

5 star	76%
4 star	9%
3 star	6%
2 star	9%
1 star	0%

˅ How customer reviews and ratings work

Review this product
Share your thoughts with other customers

Write a customer review

SCAN OR TOUCH ME

CHAPTER 5
STRONG TO THE CORE
A GROUP OF CORE EXERCISES

These exercises will help develop strength in your core muscles which help keep balance while standing. Core muscles also help minimize spinal pressure when bending, twisting, or performing reaching movements. Here are a few exercises to train your core:

EXERCISE 24: TIGHTROPE WALK

This exercise does not require special instruments and can easily be done at home. All you have to do is

- If Possible lay a straight line of duck tape on the floor, about 10-15ft.
- Extend your arms from your sides, parallel to the floor
- Walk-in a straight line, pausing every time you lift a foot off the ground for one to two seconds
- Concentrate on a distant object to keep your head straight and retain your equilibrium
- Complete 15 to 20 steps with these instructions before going on to the next exercise

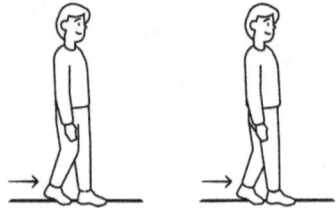

Benefits of Tightrope Walk

Provides a Full-Body Workout

When you balance yourself in a straight line, you must engage your muscles and use your entire body. The most effective and correct technique needs you to keep your lower body still and move from your hips. Use every muscle in your body to maintain your equilibrium, and you will learn to disperse your weight.

Strengthens Core

Walking on a tightrope will help you improve your core. You'll have to activate your core consistently when you're on the line, even if it doesn't appear. When you contract your core, you ensure that you are focused and well-balanced, as your body must limit excessive movements.

Improves Balance

Balance is crucial in every element of our lives, and having a good balance will benefit you later in life. It requires a lot of coordination and balance to stay upright during this exercise.

Improves Posture

Tightrope walking improves posture in older adults. Although the core muscles are the major muscle group used, the back muscles also improve your spine, ultimately improving your posture.

Enhances concentration

When effectively performing tightrope walking, you must provide your undivided attention. Practicing daily will increase your focus and give you more control over your mind's wandering thoughts. Increased concentration benefits your day-to-day activities, such as work or other activities you enjoy.

EXERCISE 25: FLAMINGO STANCE

The flamingo stance is a relatively simple and easy workout. It's what it exactly sounds like...stand like a flamingo. Follow the below-given step-by-step instructions.

- Stand on your right foot and shift your weight on it.
- Extend your left leg forward by lifting your left foot.

- Stay in this position for ten to fifteen seconds.
- You can make it more challenging by stretching your hands toward your outstretched foot.
- Shake out your legs and return to the starting posture.
- Repeat three times more.
- Then repeat on the other side.

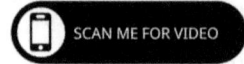

SCAN ME FOR VIDEO

Once you've mastered it, try extending your leg forward without allowing it to contact the ground or balancing without using a chair.

Practicing flamingo while standing in line or doing dishes is always a good idea. The flamingo exercise requires greater cognitive effort and burns more calories if you are new to working out. Here are some instructions on how to improve your technique:

Remove the Socks

Concentrate on distributing your weight via the heel and midfoot. Going barefoot is more effective because it boosts the stimulus to the brain and allows you to feel the floor.

Hold Your Ear

Touching your ear can keep you on your feet if you feel like you're about to fall over. Your ear is your center of balance, and touching it will re-center you.

VISUALIZE BEING ANCHORED

Imagine holding on to a bar or any other solid structure, and you might find it easier to keep your one-footed stance.

EXERCISE 26: THE SUPERMAN EXERCISE

The superman exercise is an excellent workout for people of all fitness levels. It focuses on your lower back, glutes, hamstrings, and abs muscles.

Furthermore, it complements other core work-outs that primarily target the abdominal muscles in the front of your body, such as leg raises and sit-ups.

SCAN ME FOR VIDEO

However, you might wonder how to do it effec-tively and safely to ensure you're targeting the right muscles while avoiding injury. Even if you don't become a superhero after completing this workout, you'll have a tremendously strong core after incorporating it into your training program.

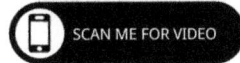

Here is how you can do this exercise:

- Lie on the ground in a facedown position with your legs straight, and arms extended.
- Slowly lift your arms and legs 6 inches off the floor or until you feel your lower back muscles contracting while keeping your head neutral (avoid looking up).
- At the same time, engage your glutes, core, and the muscles between your shoulder blades.
- To contract your abs, lift your belly button slightly off the floor.
- To visualize this, imagine yourself as Superman flying through the air.
- Maintain this posture for a few seconds.
- Make sure you're breathing throughout.
- Return to the floor by lowering your arms, legs, and belly.
- 2–3 sets of 8–12 repetitions are recommended for this workout.

It's critical to only lift as much as your body can tolerate.

You'll still get enough exercise even if you can lift a few inches off the ground. If you're having problems with this move, simply lift your arms off the ground. Also, avoid hyperextending your neck or lifting your head, which can cause pain and discomfort.

The Benefits of Superman Exercise

There are numerous advantages to the superman exercise, including:

Support for the Spine

The erector spinae muscles, which support your spine, are strengthened by this exercise.

Posture

Postural anomalies such as kyphosis ("hunchback"), which can cause poor posture and discomfort, can be prevented by having strong back muscles.

Preventing Injuries

A strong core is necessary to avoid lower back strain, which can cause pain and injury over time.

Accessibility

There is no need for any equipment for this workout; your body and the floor are all you need. As a result, it is a cost-effective exercise for everyone.

The superman exercise is practical, accessible, economical, and simple to practice for all fitness levels. That's why it's a good idea to incorporate it into your daily routine.

EXERCISE 27: SIDE BENDS

We love seated side bends because they are so simple to do. For people with mobility issues, side bends are an accessible move that still helps engage the oblique muscles on the sides of the abdomen. This can assist seniors in maintaining their balance and strengthening their ability to bend over.

SCAN ME FOR VIDEO

To do a seated side bend, follow these steps:

- Sit in a chair and place your feet flat on the floor.
- Keep one hand behind your head while reaching for the floor with the other.
- Tighten the oblique muscles on your side by leaning to the side. It is as if you're about to touch the ground.
- Return to the beginning posture after bending as far as you can and holding for three breaths.
- Repeat the same on the opposite side.

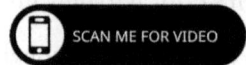

If exercising in a group, you could also have your partner do a seated twist simultaneously. They'll rotate their upper body to the left and right instead of bending to the side to work the same oblique muscles. It's a less complicated maneuver, but it's just as effective.

EXERCISE 28: WOOD CHOPS

Wood chops are a fantastic core exercise that works practically every muscle in your body while also testing your balance. It also resembles our daily tasks: filling and unloading the dishwasher.

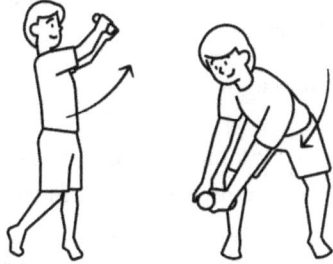

How to go about it:

- Clutch both hands in front of you with your feet wider than shoulder-width apart.
- Pull your arms up to one side of your head and hold them there.
- Squat down while maintaining your abs braced and "chopping" your arms diagonally down toward the other side of your body.
- Repeat by "chopping" your way back to the top.
- Before rotating to the other side, complete ten reps on one side.

The Benefits of doing a wood chop

This practical exercise has many advantages as it simultaneously involves multiple muscles in your trunk, hips, and shoulders.

A variety of resistance equipment, such as dumbbells, can also be used in this exercise, but are not needed.

Things to Consider Before Doing a Wood Chop

- Keep your trunk stable during this exercise. During the chopping motion, the spine tends to flex or bend forward, putting a more significant strain on your spine.
- Begin with less weight than you believe you will require to complete this workout. As needed, increase the weight while keeping adequate control.

- Reduce your range of motion and lessen your speed if you experience pain while executing this action. You can also reduce the amount of resistance applied. Stop and consult a healthcare expert if you're still in pain.

Experiment with different types of wood chops

There are many techniques to provide diversity and vary the movement's difficulty.

Stance

- Complete this exercise from a half-kneeling (lunge) stance.
- Begin with one leg in front of you and your back knee firmly beneath your hips.
- On the lead-leg side, lift the weight from the outside of your back. Keep your hip up and over to the outside of your head.

This exercise can also be done with your knees parallel to each other in a full kneeling position.

Changing the Equipment

Replace the weight with a medicine ball or kettlebell. They give diversity to the task by varying hand position and grip.

Changing the difficulty level

Bring your feet or knees closer, narrowing your support base and making the exercise more challenging. As a result, lateral instability will grow, and your muscles must work harder to maintain balance while executing the activity. Widening your posture, on the other hand, reduces the difficulty.

You can also alter the amount of weight or resistance you employ. If you go heavier, make sure you can handle the weight and aren't causing so much resistance that you have to rotate your spine excessively.

Finally, alter the speed at which you perform the movement by thinking slower for a more difficult challenge. Maintain a controlled speed while lowering the weight and carefully returning it to the beginning position, whether using a cable machine or a resistance band.

EXERCISE 29: DEAD BUG EXERCISE

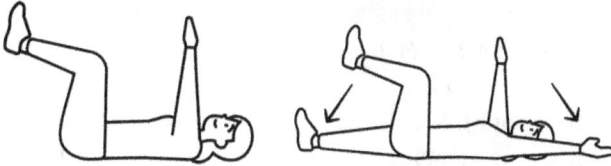

Sit-ups, crunches, reverse crunches, or even twists are likely to come to mind when thinking of core or abdominal exercises.

The dead bug exercise is also a core strengthening exercise. The problem is that the "dead bug" sounds like a disgusting or strange activity. It's not true at all. It's a simple movement that you perform while resting on your back. You extend and retract opposing extremities while keeping your chest steady and your core tight. You don't need many instruments to get started with this exercise. It's a bodyweight exercise that only requires a yoga mat. Incorporate it into your regular core-training regimen or after a cardio workout.

Step-by-Step Instructions

The dead bug exercise is done on the ground, so you should usually utilize a yoga mat or another workout mat for added comfort.

- Lie down on the mat.
- Keep your arms straight across your chest, forming a perpendicular angle with your torso.
- Take your feet off the ground and bend your hips and knees 90 degrees.
- Your torso and thighs, as well as your thighs and shins, should make a perfect angle. This is where it all begins.
- Engage your core to keep your lower back in contact with the mat.
- Make sure your spine stays stable and neutral throughout the workout
- Maintain the position of your right arm and left leg, then reach your left arm backward, over your head, and toward the floor while simultaneously extending your right knee and hip, reaching your right heel toward the floor.

- As you complete the extensions, move gently and firmly, breathing in and out, avoiding any twisting or movement of your hips and abs.
- Come to a complete stop before your arm and leg touch the ground.
- Now return your left arm and right leg to the initial positions by reversing the movement. Exhale as you move gently and steadily.
- Carry through the identical actions on the other side, but keep your left arm and right leg still.
- Do the same number of repetitions on each side.

Benefits

The exercise strengthens the core muscles of the body. The abs are an essential part of your overall core musculature, encompassing all muscle groups that run from your hips to your shoulders. These muscles operate together to convey movement between your upper and lower bodies, anchor the spine, and keep it from shifting unnaturally. As a result, a strong, stable core can help you move more smoothly and athletically while preventing your lower back from injury.

The dead bug is an effective exercise for increasing opposing limb activation while promoting overall core stability. This essentially implies that the exercise teaches you to move opposing limbs in synchrony while maintaining your core and back safe.

The dead bug is a beginner-friendly technique that allows you to acclimate to contralateral limb extension while maintaining core stability and protection. The dead bug promotes the deep, stabilizing muscles of your low back, abdominals, and hips to engage during the exercise, preventing your back from twisting or arching. You'll improve side-to-side coordination and deep core strength, which can help you avoid low-back injuries.

The dead bug is an excellent alternative for those who aren't quite ready for the more well-known plank exercise. Both movements are meant to help with core stabilization, but the plank might be challenging for people who don't have a lot of core strength or have low back problems. The dead bug can help with core stabilization while adding the challenge of contra-lateral limb movement to the plank.

Common Mistakes While Performing Dead Bug Exercise

Moving Too Quickly

A common mistake people make with the dead bug exercise is to confuse it with a bicycle crunch and try to propel themselves through using speed and momentum.You've made this mistake if you see your extremities moving simultaneously—as if you haven't come to a complete halt at the top of the movement before beginning the action to the opposite side.

We all have heard that slow and steady wins the race. The same is the case with stability. Slow down even more if you fear you're going too quickly. Your torso shifts as you start gaining speed, and you lose your core's ideal steadiness.

If you can't stop yourself from speeding through each rep, grab a stability ball or a foam roller and place it between your hands and knees as you prepare to begin the exercise. The goal is to keep the instrument from falling, which you won't be able to do if you use more than two extremities at once. You must slow down and "reset" between each repeat before continuing the exercise on the opposing side by keeping it in place with one hand and one knee as your opposite extremities expand.

Arching Lower Back Away from the Floor

Due to weak core stabilizers, your back may automatically arch up and away from the floor when completing supine abdominal workouts. Your low back muscles aren't strong enough to keep it in place.

If you find your back arching, slow down and try to remedy the problem. If slowing down doesn't help, try the trick of holding a stability ball or foam roller steady with two limbs as the opposite extremities move through their extensions, as described above.

Reduce the range of your extensions if you still can't keep your low back from arching off the floor. Only extend your leg and the contralateral arm as far as your spine will allow without arching. Bring your arm and leg back to center when you feel your low back arching, then repeat on the opposite side.

Variations of Dead Bugs Exercise

The dead bug exercise is a relatively simple movement, but anyone with weak core stabilizers may have trouble maintaining perfect form. If you're having trouble keeping your body still while performing the dead bug, try moving one extremity at a time rather than opposing arms and legs.

Instead of simultaneously extending your right arm and left leg, consider extending your right arm alone. Extend your left leg after bringing it back to the center. Do the same thing with your left arm and right leg when you've brought your left leg back to the center.

Try the opposite arm-opposite leg challenge again once you can move each extremity independently, but change the range of motion accordingly, halting your extensions when you feel your torso shift or your low back arch off the floor.

How to Make this Exercise More Challenging?

Add weight to the basic dead bug. As you extend your contra-lateral limbs, hold a lightweight dumbbell in each hand or hook a resistance band between your opposite hand and foot to increase resistance. If you're using a resistance band, make sure you finish all of the reps on one side before switching.

Precautions and Safety

For the most part, the dead bug is a safe activity for most people. The most significant risk of injury, like with any strengthening action, occurs when you forgo good form to "gut out" a series of repetitions. Just keep in mind that it's your ego talking.

If your form begins to deteriorate, your muscles are most likely exhausted, and it's time to end your set. Increasing the number of repetitions while maintaining bad technique will not aid your efforts to become stronger and may even result in injury, particularly to the low back.

Slow down and focus on form first—make sure your low back isn't arching and your body isn't moving back and forth as you move. Second, don't force yourself to complete the movement if it hurts if you know you have a lower-back problem. Sharp or jabbing aches or any discomfort that makes you think, "I won't be able to move tomorrow," are what you want to avoid.

If the dead bug isn't working for you, talk to a trainer or physical therapist about other possibilities.

EXERCISE 30: PLANK

The abdominal and core muscles are numerous layered muscle groups that work together to keep us upright and preserve our spine and internal organs.

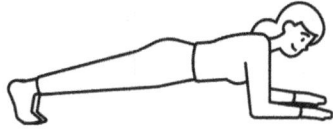

Weak abdominal muscles can lead to various issues, including mild lower back pain, hernias, chronic back pain, and a higher chance of injury during vigorous activity and hobbies.

Strong abdominal muscles are necessary for maintaining balance in walking, lifting objects, and carrying out daily tasks.

However, there are some risks that older individuals should be aware of when doing abdominal workouts. The fundamental reason is that our spines degrade and become less mobile as we age. The intervertebral discs compress, and the vertebrae fuse to prevent excessive movement that could irritate or harm the nerves. You might aggravate these fusion structures by performing abdominal motions like ab crunches or leg lifts that involve spinal flexion.

However, if you cannot undertake ab workouts, how can you improve your abdominal muscles? Of course, with planks!

What exactly is a plank?

Plank is a stability exercise that focuses primarily on the abdominal muscles. In truth, it works the entire body practically, making it a highly effective and functional exercise.

The plank is performed in a fixed position since it is an isometric exercise. Your muscles strive against gravity to keep you in that position.

Although the notion may appear simple, performing an entire plank demands significant strength.

But how can you include increasing difficulty into a static isometric exercise? There are a couple of approaches.

The first is a series of movement modifications of varying degrees of difficulty. Planks can be made more difficult by increasing leverage, exactly like push-ups. It's best to start on your knees and work your way up to a complete plank.

The second option is to add time to the equation. While increasing isometric contraction time isn't the most effective approach to increasing muscular strength, it's ideal for the abdominals.

This is because the main job of the abdominals is to be able to firmly contract when you need to brace your midsection (like lifting something heavy).

Adding time to the plank will strengthen the bracing pattern while allowing you to hold it for extended periods. Making it more likely that your abs will protect your spine during strenuous activities and light exercise.

Variations in Planks

There are various ways to do planks to target different core sections with varying degrees of difficulty. The general guideline is that the greater the distance between your support points (forearms vs. feet), the more complex the variation.

There are three valuable plank variants for seniors

Kneeling Plank

Because of the shorter leverage, the modified plank on the knees is easier to complete. It is carried out as follows:

- Begin on your elbows and knees on the floor.
- Lift your torso and hips off the floor while clenching your abdominals.
- Maintain a comfortable low hip position.
- Make sure to engage your abs and keep your spine neutral.

The Standard Plank

The conventional plank is far more challenging to do than the plank on the knees. Because you must support your entire body weight between your feet and elbows, your legs and hips are more active in this form.

It's called a plank because the goal is to keep your body as straight as a plank, so keep your back and hips straight.

- You begin on your elbows and toes on the floor.

- Lift your body, hips, and knees off the floor while clenching your abdominals.
- Maintain a comfortable low hip position.
- Engage your abs, and keep your spine in a neutral position.

The plank becomes significantly more challenging because of a substantial body weight to support and additional muscles.

Side Plank

The side plank is the final variation. As the name implies, it's done on your side. Side planks should not be attempted until you have mastered the standard plank variations. The side planks activate the obliques.

This is since gravity will naturally unilaterally affect you when you are sideways. In a plank, the most taxed muscles are closest to the ground. As a result, if you do a side plank on your right side, your right-side obliques will have to work the hardest to support your body weight. This isn't to say they're the only muscles involved. Quite the opposite is true. Most of your body muscles are used as stabilizers in the plank.

To perform a side plank lay parallel to the ground. Slowly place your forearm on the floor and lift your body weight using your feet. Raise your non based arm straight into the air.

Muscles targeted during planks

As previously stated, planks engage most of your body's muscles to stabilize your trunk while maintaining an isometric contraction.

The most significant muscle groups during this exercise are the abdominal and spinal erectors, which keep your spine from overextending as you maintain the plank.

Are planks beneficial for senior citizens?

Planks are particularly beneficial to seniors since they are the only effective abdominal and core workout that does not involve spinal flexion and extension. This implies less danger of worsening or causing new lower back problems. The core muscles are the most crucial aspect of your spinal health for back pain.

Strong core muscles protect your spine from injuries and poor posture, contributing to further degeneration and back pain. The core muscles are needed for almost every action, such as standing or walking. These muscles are essential for balance and strength training. Tennis, running, kayaking, and weight training requires specific core strength to perform safely and successfully. Planks will aid you in your endeavor.

Planks are a type of strength training.Therefore, they'll help you get all the health benefits of strength training.

A strong core will also aid in maintaining good posture and squeezing your waistline. Don't we all want to look and live our best?

EXERCISE 31: SCISSOR KICKS

The scissor kick is one of many exercises that you may use to strengthen and maintain your core. It also works your lower body and requires you to employ several muscles to complete the task. Flutter kicks is another name for this exercise.

SCAN ME FOR VIDEO

- Begin by lying on your back with your arms by your sides. Keep your palms down, pressing into the ground for support.
- Maintain a flat lower back by bracing your abs and keeping your lower back flat against the floor.
- Raise both legs to a 45-degree angle from the floor, keeping them straight.
- Then lower one leg to the floor while elevating the other over your hips.
- Now start switching your legs up and down in a scissor motion.
- If your lower back arches away from the floor during this exercise, you'll need to start with more straightforward lower abdominal exercises to strengthen your core.

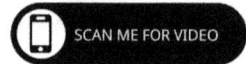

EXERCISE 32: ROLL-UPS (ADVANCED)

One of the most common pilates mat exercises is the roll-up. It is an excellent test for the abdominal muscles. One Pilates roll-up is considered to be equivalent to six ordinary sit-ups and is far superior to crunches for achieving a flat stomach.

While rolling up is one of the first mat exercises you will learn, it is difficult, and you may need to adjust it or increase your core strength before you can execute it correctly.

- Lie down on your back with your arms and legs stretched out in front of you.
- Bring your arms aloft and slowly curl your upper body off the floor as you inhale.
- Continue to slide forward until you reach your toes.
- Then, as you exhale, reverse the movement, letting one vertebra at a time rest on the ground.
- Repeat the same for 45 seconds and then rest for a few seconds.

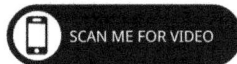

Benefits of Roll-Ups

The Pilates Roll Up has several advantages. This exercise activates your spine and builds your abdominal muscles by putting them through various motions. The roll-up is an effective exercise for building core strength, stability, and muscular endurance. These advantages will carry over into your regular life, enhancing your ability to execute lifting and bending chores while protecting your spine. You'll also be less likely to fall and get hurt.

EXERCISE 33: STRAIGHT LEG RAISES

Leg workout activities help strengthen the lower body, promoting balance and flexibility. As a result, functional independence and confidence rise. Press your back onto the floor when your straight leg rises. This aligns your spine, which improves your safety and comfort.

The exercise also strengthens your quadriceps, hip flexors, and abdominal muscles. The exercise allows you to walk with greater ease by allowing you to advance your leg. Give it a try.

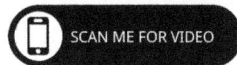

- Lay on your back with one knee bent and the other straight, toes pointing to the ceiling.
- Raise your straightened leg to the same level as the bent knee on the other side.
- Return to the beginning pose and repeat the same ten times more with each leg.
- Inhale during the upward movement phase.
- Exhale during the downward movement phase.

To gain greater support:

1. Place your palms down.
2. During the lifting portion, exhale.
3. Do not lift one knee higher than the other.

Take it to the next step.

Place a 2 to 5lb weight on your ankle for this leg workout. For ten seconds, stay in the raised position.

CHAPTER 6
WATCH YOUR STEP
A GROUP OF WALKING EXERCISES

Walking works wonders for seniors! Regular aerobic activity, such as walking, provides numerous health benefits for older individuals. Walking as a form of exercise has several benefits, including relief from arthritis symptoms, reduced anxiety and sadness, and improved heart health. Regarding balance, walking triggers the receptors in our feet and makes us aware of our position in space.

WHY WALK?

Walking aids in developing lower-body strength, a critical component of excellent balance. Walking is a healthy form of exercise for active older adults, and it contributes to your aerobic activity objectives and improves balance. If you have health issues that make walking difficult, your doctor or physical therapist can advise you on additional possibilities.

Whether you're sedentary or moderately active, an intelligent walking strategy should be intended to increase physical activity safely. The minutes, not the miles, are what matters. Here's how to make a walking plan that's right for you:

Start from the beginning if you haven't been exercising. Make sure you use a cane or walker if you regularly do so. Increase the length of your walks as you become more robust and comfortable.

Things to consider before you start walking exercises

Start Smart

Choosing a realistic strategy and sticking to it is the key to a successful walking program. Don't get too carried away. The advantages of walking accrue over time. Make sure your time and energy output are acceptable for your age and health. According to the Centers for Disease Control and Prevention, older individuals should exercise moderately to mildly for at least 2.5 hours each week. For seven days, that equates to around 20 minutes per day. This advice, however, is not a hard and fast rule. Choose what works best for you and start walking at your own pace.

Warming Up

Warm up your muscles and perform a balance check before beginning a strenuous walking routine. Begin with small steps. Raise your arms above your head and stand up tall. Rotate your arms in a windmill motion if you're feeling stable. This increases blood flow and relaxes your arm and shoulder muscles. Stand behind a chair and hang on to it with one hand if you're feeling unsteady. Lift one foot at a time, then the other. This gentle balance practice can help you get ready to start walking.

Setting the Pace

Know where you're heading before you start. Start slowly and choose a path that you're familiar with. For beginners, the flat and broad surfaces are the best. As you walk, use your complete body, including your arms. Slowly swing your arms back and forth; don't overdo it; it shouldn't hurt. When you add arm mobility to your walking regimen, you engage your entire body and increase your aerobic benefits. Set a reasonable pace, and allow at least 5 to 10 minutes at that rate before beginning to push yourself.

The Road to Power Walking

A regular and consistent walking regimen can be a foundation for a more intensive aerobic and strength-training program. You can start integrating more components in your walking program once you've learned your capabilities. Strength training is a simple one to incorporate. Begin holding a 1 to 2lb weight in each hand during your walks. The weights mustn't feel overly heavy. Attempt to lift each weight eight to ten times. If this is not a difficult task, the weight is appropriate for you. If you can't lift it, the weight is too heavy. Once you've got it down, go for a stroll with your hand weights, lifting them with your strides along your usual route for a wonderful full-body workout.

Engage Body and Mind

Walking boosts your overall system and can be essential to living a healthy and independent senior life. Be reasonable and practical while beginning your walking regimen for the best results. The goal is to reap the advantages of exercise while knowing your limits and being acquainted with your own body.

Here we have discussed a few walking exercises that will help you improve balance and mobility. Follow the guide for each exercise mentioned here.

EXERCISE 34: WALKING IN PLACE

As the name implies, walking in place is raising the knees in a walking motion while remaining stationary. This exercise is convenient since you can do it anywhere—at a standing desk at work, in line at the shop, on the sidelines of your child's soccer game, etc.

Walking in place is not to be confused with walking around your house, which entails walking about your home. Both of these activities are examples of indoor walking. On the other hand, House walking involves traveling from one spot to another. When you walk in place you stay in the same spot. You can use walking in place to stay active while watching TV at home. You can also walk-in place while cooking dinner standing beside the stove. You may even walk-in place in the open air if you need to let your dog out; walk-in place until you can let him back in. You can walk-in place while your children play outside, ensuring they are safe and having fun.

The Best Way to Walk in Place

Follow these instructions to start walking in place.

- Put on your walking shoes and start walking. While walking in place for a few minutes without shoes may be acceptable, you should put on a pair of walking shoes if you plan to stroll longer. This provides the necessary support for your feet.

- Begin walking. It's as easy as it sounds. Get up and start walking in place the next time you find yourself sitting. You can walk in place independently or while multitasking. Are you waiting for the oven timer to beep? Laundry folding? Are you on the phone? Do you like to watch television? To any of these, add walking in place!
- Keep track of your steps. Motivation is crucial. Seeing how many steps you can take with a pedometer, or using the health app on your phone or watch, will motivate you to walk in place whenever feasible.
- Make a step target for yourself. Each day, try to walk a specified number of steps. Step it up once you've met your step goal for a few days.
- Use a heart rate monitor to keep track of your progress. A monitor can help determine whether walking in place raises your heart rate sufficiently to improve your cardiovascular health.
- You can use a heart rate monitor to ensure you're in your goal heart rate zone. Swing your arms more or lift your legs higher if you need to step it up a notch.

Do intervals

Is the thought of strolling in place a little too boring for you? Instead of walking at the same pace the entire time, increase your speed for a minute or two before lowering it. You've now completed an interval training session by alternating between faster and slower paces.

Add strength training moves

Including muscle-building motions in your walking routine can turn it into a total-body workout. This is where bodyweight workouts come in handy. Do a few push-ups after a few minutes of walking in place. Continue walking in place for a few minutes more, then do a few crunches. You'll have worked for every muscle group in your body by the time you're done!

There are still methods to keep ourselves active and strive toward a healthier lifestyle despite our hectic schedules. One approach that can help you do both is to walk in place.

EXERCISE 35: TANDEM WALK WITH BALL TOSS

Dual-task performance, or when a person's attention is split between a motor and a cognitive task, is typical in everyday life. Under mental stress or when engaged in attention-demanding tasks, healthy older people and those with balance impairments show lower physical performance, increasing the chance of falling.

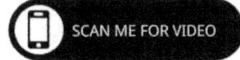

SCAN ME FOR VIDEO

Balance training in dual-task scenarios is essential to increase balance control in situations requiring divided attention. A tandem walk with a ball toss is a dual-task exercise that improves your balance. Follow the below-given instructions for this exercise.

- Stand up straight with a clear path in front of you.
- Imagine a straight line stretching away from you on the floor, or tape a straight line across the floor.
- Walk along this line on the floor as if you were walking a tightrope,
- While walking in a straight path, throw a tennis ball into the air and catch it again.
- Try to maintain your balance while catching the ball and avoid falling.
- Make sure to toss the ball above eye level.

EXERCISE 36: BACKWARD STEPS

We move forward every day, so when we fall in that direction, our bodies instinctively know what to do: step or reach to stop ourselves. However, if the older adult's balance is lost backward, they will usually react in one of two ways:

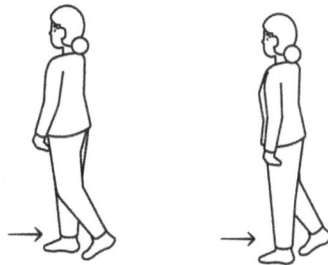

Indecision, anxiety and or fear immobilizes them for a bit of a moment, then a painful drop toward the floor ensues.

Or they take a series of quick, little steps backward, attempting to keep up with their momentum until they can't.

The motion is usually stopped by a counter, wall, chair, or floor.

The body learns familiarity with the action and is prepared to react to the movement to avoid a backwards fall by practicing taking steps backward.

- Standing at the counter, take a single step backward, shifting your weight to your rear foot, and stop.
- Add tilting forward at the hips as you step back once that is fluid and easy. This quickly shifts weight, making it more difficult for the body to continue going rearward into a fall.
- Here is the guide on how to practice walking backward safely.
- The most fantastic idea is to find a wall where you can take at least ten steps in a row with the wall remaining next to you
- Begin by stepping backward while holding on to the wall with one hand.
- Return to your starting place by turning around and walking backward.
- Repeat this process four times more. That is all there is to it. This activity is fantastic for improving your balance.
- As you walk, try to keep your eyes up.
- If you're afraid to do this exercise, make sure you're accompanied by someone to keep you safe.
- Why not try this workout a few times a week because it is simple and beneficial to your balance? As you go about your everyday activities, you will notice a significant improvement in your balance.

EXERCISE 37: STANDING MARCH WITH ARMS

The standing march is an exercise that is recommended for seniors who want to improve their balance. Cross your arms in front of your chest and hold them there. Raise one of your knees toward your arms at a time.

Contralateral Marching

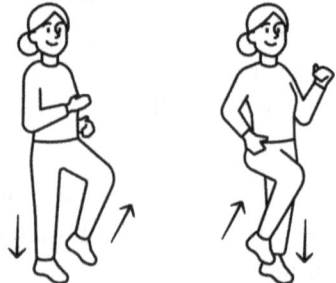

- Raise the right arm to any height overhead while simultaneously lifting the left leg to a 90-degree angle at the hip.
- Return to the starting position after three to five seconds.
- Raise the left arm overhead and the right leg to 90 degrees simultaneously.
- Train alternate sides as needed

Ipsilateral Marching

- Ipsilateral marching involves raising the right arm above the head while simultaneously raising the right leg at the hip to 90 degrees.
- Lower to the starting position after three to five seconds of holding.
- Raise the left arm overhead while lifting the left leg to a 90-degree angle at the hip.

EXERCISE 38: SIDE STEP CLAPS

- Stand up with your back straight and your feet together.
- Raise your elbows in front of your body.
- Bring elbows together at shoulder height.
- Close palms of hands together and bend elbows at a 90-degree angle.
- Alternate side steps, taking two to the right and two to the left while gently bending your knees.
- As you take a stride to the side, open your elbows and bring your elbows and feet back together.
- Maintain a low shoulder position and a straight back.
- Do this exercise for two sets of 30 seconds each.
- Between each set, take a 30-second break.
- Work at a level appropriate for your physical capabilities, boosting your cardiovascular system's production.
- Don't push yourself too much.

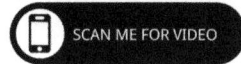

SCAN ME FOR VIDEO

Let me make it simple for you. Begin by standing with your feet together and your hands by your sides. Swing your arms to the side as you hop out to the right with your right leg. Step with your left leg together and clap at the same time. Now, with your left leg, leap out to the left. Bring your right leg in to meet your left and clap together.

EXERCISE 39: HEEL-TO-TOE WALK

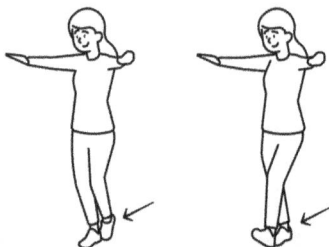

There are many great activities you can do to enhance your balance. One of these is the heel-toe walk. This workout helps to strengthen your legs while also improving your balance. The heel-toe walk, also known as the tandem walk, is simple to master in any scenario where you can take 4-8 consecutive steps forward and back. Start by walking along a kitchen counter or wall with one hand on the surface to ensure your safety. exercise with both arms dangling at your sides in an open place as you progress.

- Clear your walking path of any carpets and other obstacles to avoid tripping hazards.
- Stand with a healthy upright posture against a wall with your heels pressed on it.
- Your left foot should be in front of your right foot.
- Make a connection between your left heel and your right toes.
- Then, step forward with your right foot in front of your left.
- Make a connection between your right heel and your left toes.
- Maintain a clear view of the horizon.
- Examine the floor and the area around you with your peripheral vision. This ability allows you to walk without having to look down.
- Imagine walking on a tightrope and placing one foot in front of the other. If this is too difficult, switch to a semi-tandem position.
- You can gently offset the forward foot's heel from the rear foot's toes instead of placing it precisely in front of them.
- Step backward and return to the starting position after 4-8 steps forward, depending on your space.

- Do the heel-toe walk back and forth multiple times a day to maintain your feet on the ground and walk confidently.
- Continue for a total of 20 steps.

How to make this exercise more challenging?

- Raise your arms to your sides and hold them there.
- As you continue, you can cross your hands over your chest.
- This arm position makes the heel-toe walk exercise more challenging.
- Another good alternative is to practice the heel-toe walk while holding a weighted ball (near to your body).

EXERCISE 40: SERPENTINE WALK

Every time you change directions, your body will need to rebalance.

SCAN ME FOR VIDEO

- You can do this by walking a figure eight around two spots at least five feet apart or by zigzagging back and forth as if you were doing a slalom run-around cones.
- Walk three steps to one side of the walkway, then switch to angling to the other side for three steps.
- Repeat the process numerous times.

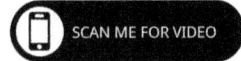

This is a valuable method to adopt when downhill traveling and generating your little switchbacks.

Check Your Posture Before You Begin

It's critical to have a good walking posture to improve your balance. Suck in your stomach, tuck in your behind, and twist your hips slightly forward as you stand straight, shoulders back and relaxed, chin parallel to the ground, gaze forward. There should be no forward or backward leaning, and your back should not be arched.

EXERCISE 41: BALANCE WALK

Good balance allows you to move safely while avoiding tripping and falling over obstacles. There is a halt while on one foot throughout the walk. It adds to the difficulty of this balance exercise.

SCAN ME FOR VIDEO

- Begin with your arms spread out at shoulder height from your sides.
- Concentrate on a location several feet ahead of you with your chin up and not looking at the ground.
- Start walking. Lift your back leg and bring it forward, pausing with your knee up before stepping forward with your foot on the ground.
- Carry on with the opposite leg in the same manner.
- Pause for a second with your knee up before placing that foot ahead of you as you draw it forward.
- Repeat for a total of 20 steps.
- Try looking from side to side as you walk as you progress, but if you have inner ear problems, avoid this step.
- If you're feeling shaky, try doing this exercise close to a wall or with someone nearby to help you.

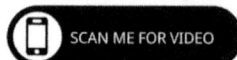

FINAL WORDS ABOUT WALKING EXERCISES

Walking was formerly the only mode of transportation available to humanity. We had to rely on our two feet to move from one point to another. As time progressed, we discovered new means to travel around more swiftly. But this easiness led to many other health problems. When going to the grocery store these days, most individuals look for the closest parking spot to the door to prevent a long walk inside.

On the other hand, walking has many advantages, particularly for seniors. Including at least 30 minutes of daily walking in your routine helps you avoid a sedentary lifestyle and benefits your health.

Benefits of walking exercises for seniors

According to experts, walking is the best exercise for seniors since it improves balance, reduces the risk of chronic illnesses, and improves general health. The following are some of the advantages of walking exercises for seniors. Each walking exercise:

It improves cardiovascular health

Walking exercises have several heart health benefits for elders. Daily increasing your heart rate lowers your risk of hypertension, high cholesterol, and even coronary heart disease.

Reduces blood sugar levels

A 15-minute stroll after eating has been demonstrated to minimize the after-meal blood sugar increase that some seniors suffer. Your body utilizes blood sugar to develop muscles, and insulin works better.

Pain reduction

Studies have found walking helps alleviate pain associated with chronic illnesses such as arthritis. Lower back pain affects many seniors, and walking for 20 minutes three times a week might help strengthen stomach and back muscles, reducing chronic back pain.

Cost-free exercises

You can perform walking exercises at almost any place for free once you've invested in a nice, solid pair of sneakers. When the weather permits, take a walk around your neighborhood. You can also go to the park for a stroll down the route. If the weather is too chilly or rainy to go outside, try walking in place indoors instead.

Encourages social interaction

Whether you join a walking group with pals or connect with neighbors while on your daily walk, walking is an easy opportunity for seniors to meet up with others. Walking is an excellent opportunity to meet new people and enjoy your surroundings.

Enhances mental well-being

A daily walk might make you feel better about yourself and your life. Endorphins, released during physical activity, provide a feeling of well-being, reduce anxiety, and improve mood.

HOW TO INCORPORATE WALKING INTO YOUR DAILY ROUTINE?

The fundamental purpose of a rehabilitation program is to get patients back on their feet and walking. Patients are encouraged to get out of bed and walk after hip replacement surgery to increase blood circulation and prevent muscles and joints from stiffening. It's a low-impact way for seniors to strengthen their muscles and bones while improving cardio-vascular fitness.

Start reaping the benefits of walking by including it in your daily routine. Get a pair of durable, supportive sneakers, lace them up, and then choose a known, obstacle-free path. To relieve joint strain, make sure the surface is smooth and soft. Begin with a 10-minute stroll and progressively increase the duration and speed of your walk. Dress for the weather, and don't forget to drink plenty of water! If you have any pain while walking, stop and take a rest; if the pain persists, see your doctor.

CHAPTER 7
VERTI-GO AWAY!
A GROUP OF VESTIBULAR EXERCISES

A sensation of spinning and dizziness characterizes vertigo. It can be a sign of various other problems. The condition can occur when there is a problem with the inner ear, brain, or sensory nerve route.

Dizziness, including vertigo, can strike anyone at any age, but it is more common in persons over 65. People can have vertigo for a short time or for a long time. It can happen during pregnancy or indicate a bacterial infection in the ear. Vertigo can occur in people with inner ear problems, such as Meniere's disease.

Continue reading this chapter to learn more about vertigo, including the various causes, treatments, and exercises that can help restore the lost balance.

Vertigo is a common condition. A person may feel like the room or surroundings are whirling in circles. Although this is not always right, the phrase is frequently used to indicate a fear of heights. When a person stares down from a considerable height, vertigo might arise. However, the term vertigo is more commonly used to describe any momentary or continuous dizziness caused by inner ear or brain issues. Vertigo itself is not a disease but a symptom of an underlying problem. There can be various causes of vertigo.

INNER EAR ISSUES

A network of tubes filled with fluid runs through the inner ear. These canals are tilted at various angles. As the head moves, the movement of the fluid inside it tells the brain how far, fast, and in which direction it is moving. The brain then uses this information to move the eyes in the opposite direction, ensuring that the image the eyes see does not blur and remains clear. Here are a few common inner ear problems that can cause vertigo.

1. Labyrinthitis

Dizziness, spinning sensations (vertigo), and balance issues are all symptoms of labyrinthitis, an inner ear illness. Labyrinthitis is caused by inner ear infections and other ear disorders. The most common cause of labyrinthitis is a virus or bacterial infection. The labyrinth, a network of fluid-filled passages in the inner ear, gets inflamed during this disease. This inflammation can disrupt the transmission of sensory information from the inner ear to the brain and is responsible for the symptoms of labyrinthitis.

Prevalence of Labyrinthitis

Viral labyrinthitis most usually affects adults between the ages of 30 and 60. Women are also affected twice as often as males. Labyrinthitis is prevalent after a more common infection, such as a cold or the flu. In some circumstances, labyrinthitis is caused by a bacterial infection.

1. Vestibular Neuritis

Vestibular neuritis is an inner ear disease that can cause abrupt, severe vertigo (a spinning/swaying sensation), dizziness, balance issues, nausea, and vomiting. The condition affects the vestibulocochlear nerve, which runs through the inner ear. The inner ear delivers information regarding balance and head position via this nerve. When this nerve becomes inflamed, it causes problems with how the brain interprets information. As a result, dizziness and vertigo are common symptoms. Vestibular neuritis can affect people of all ages; however, it is uncommon in children.

Significant Symptoms of Vestibular Neuritis

- Sudden, severe vertigo (a sense of spinning or swaying)
- Dizziness
- Problems with balance
- Vomiting and nausea
- Problems with concentration

Vestibular neuritis and labyrinthitis are closely related. Vestibular neuritis is a balance disorder caused by the swelling of a branch of the vestibulo-cochlear nerve (the vestibular part). Labyrinthitis is the swelling of both branches of the vestibulocochlear nerve (the vestibular and cochlear portions), affecting balance and hearing. The symptoms of labyrinthitis are similar to those of vestibular neuritis. However, these are with the addition of tinnitus (ringing in the ear) and hearing loss.

The most severe symptoms usually only last a few days, but they make daily activities challenging while they are present. Over the next few weeks, most patients make a slow but complete recovery when the severe symptoms subside (approximately three weeks). On the other hand, some patients may experience long-term dizziness and balance problems.

Causes of Vestibular Neuritis

The most common causes are an inner ear viral infection, viral-induced swelling around the vestibulocochlear nerve, or a viral infection else-where in the body. Viral infections in various body parts include the herpes virus (which causes cold sores, shingles, and chickenpox), measles, flu, mumps, hepatitis, and polio. (Genital herpes does not induce vestibular neuritis.)

How can you know if you have vestibular neuritis?

A diagnosis of vestibular neuritis can usually be made during a visit to a vestibular specialist's clinic. An otologist (ear doctor) or a neurotologist (a doctor specializing in the nervous system related to the ear) are two professionals who can diagnose vestibular neuritis. An audiologist (hearing clinician) may be referred to conduct additional tests to assess hearing and vestibular damage.

Hearing tests, vestibular (balancing) tests, and a test to check if a segment of the vestibulocochlear nerve has been destroyed are all used to identify if symptoms are caused by vestibular neuritis. Another test, known as a head impulse test, looks at how challenging it is to retain focus on items while moving your head quickly. Vestibular neuritis is diagnosed by the presence of nystagmus or uncontrollable fast eye movement.

If symptoms persist for more than a few weeks or worsen, more tests are performed to see if other illnesses or diseases cause the symptoms. Stroke, head injury, brain tumor, and migraine headaches are other possible health conditions. An MRI using dye (called a contrast agent) may be conducted to rule out several brain diseases.

TREATMENT AND MANAGEMENT OF VESTIBULAR NEURITIS

The symptoms of vestibular neuritis are managed, a virus is treated (if diagnosed), and a balance rehabilitation program is completed.

Taking care of the symptoms

The goal of treatment for vestibular neuritis when it first appears is to alleviate symptoms. Ondansetron (Zofran) and metoclopramide (Reglan) are two anti-nausea medications. Patients may be hospitalized and given IV fluids to treat dehydration if nausea and vomiting are severe and cannot be managed with medication.

Meclizine, diazepam (Valium), and lorazepam (Ativan) are all used to treat dizziness. The many forms of dizziness-relieving medicines are grouped and referred to as vestibular suppressants. Vestibular suppressants should only be administered for three days at a time. They are not advised for long-term usage because they can make a recovery more complex. Steroids are sometimes utilized as well.

Treating the Virus

Antiviral treatment, such as acyclovir, is given if the vestibular neuritis is considered to be caused by a herpes virus. (Antibiotics aren't used to treat vestibular neuritis because it's not a bacterial infection.)

Balance Rehabilitation Program

A vestibular physical therapy program may be indicated if balance and dizziness difficulties persist for more than a few weeks. This treatment aims to train the brain to adjust to the variations in balance that a patient experiences.

As the first step in this process, a vestibular physical therapist evaluates the body components that affect balance. These are some of the areas:

Legs: How well the legs "feel" balanced when attempting to stand or walk.

Eyes: How well the sense of vision interprets the body's position in its surroundings.

Ears: How well the inner ear works to keep you balanced.

The entire body: How effectively does the body understand its center of gravity – does it sway or have an uneven posture.

Based on the evaluation results, an exercise regimen is created individually for the patient. Vestibular balance exercises are discussed next in this chapter.

BENIGN PAROXYSMAL POSITIONAL VERTIGO (BPPV)

Benign paroxysmal positional vertigo is one of the most common causes of vertigo. Each part of the name refers to a different aspect of the condition:

It's benign as it's not too serious. Your life isn't at risk.

It is paroxysmal because it occurs suddenly, lasts briefly, and comes and goes.

Positional vertigo occurs when particular postures or head motions cause dizziness.

Causes

Most of us don't know, but there are calcium carbonate crystals inside the ear. They're sometimes referred to as "ear rocks." Otoconia is another name for them.

Crystals can become dislodged from their usual location in your ear and travel to other parts of your body, including the canals in your ears that feel your head's rotation. They can gather together and form a clump. The clump will sink to the lowest area of your inner ear since it is hefty in comparison to other objects in your ear. When you turn or shift position, the clump will cause the fluid in your inner ear to slosh about after stopping moving. This gives the impression that you're moving even though you're not. Benign paroxysmal can be provoked by moving your head in a variety of ways:

- Turning over in bed
- Getting into and out of bed
- Bending over while doing yoga
- Getting your hair rinsed in a salon with your head tilted back
- Rapid head movements

When you have BPPV, you might anticipate having rhythmic eye movements. This is known as "nystagmus" by doctors, and it's what they'll look for if they suspect you have vertigo. The condition can be significant in rare situations if it makes you more likely to fall. If you're having these episodes regularly, it could signify something more serious. However, they're notoriously tricky to diagnose.

1. **Meniere's disease**

Meniere's disease is an inner-ear disease that causes dizziness (vertigo) and hearing loss. Meniere's disease usually affects one ear and can strike at any age. Young to middle-aged adults are the most affected. Although it's a chronic ailment, several therapies can assist in alleviating symptoms and reducing the long-term impact on your life.

Causes and Triggers of Meniere's Disease

Although the specific etiology of Meniere's is unknown, it is thought to be related to increased pressure in the inner ear, which is filled with a fluid called endolymph. Meniere's disease is also known as primary idiopathic endolymphatic hydrops, which refers to abnormal fluid in the inner ear. Meniere's disease can be caused by or triggered by a variety of factors, including:

- Head Injury or a history of concussions
- A bacterial infection of the inner or middle ear
- Allergies
- Use of alcoholic beverages
- Stress

- Side effects of some drugs
- Smoking
- Anxiety
- Fatigue
- A history of the disease in the family
- Infection of the lungs
- A recent viral infection
- The abnormal immune response
- Migraines

Now that we have discussed almost all causes of vertigo, let's look at the solutions to this condition.

EXERCISE 42: HEAD ROTATIONS

In instances where vision alterations are present, head rotations can aid balance. This is a simple warm-up that strengthens your neck muscles and helps you improve your balance.

SCAN ME FOR VIDEO

- Stand tall and align your feet with your hips.
- For 30 seconds, gently rotate your head from left to right and then up and down.
- Repeat the circuit, but this time in the opposite direction.
- Stop or move your head more slowly if you start to feel dizzy.
- Stop the exercise and try again later if the dizziness persists.
- You can start by practicing this exercise while sitting and gradually progress to standing.

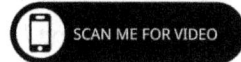

EXERCISE 43: CLOCK REACH

This exercise is especially beneficial for people who have trouble balancing due to visual or movement limitations. A chair is needed to perform this exercise. Here is how you can do it.

Assume you're in the middle of a clock. You are immediately behind the number 6 and directly in front of the number 12.

- Hold the chair with your left hand.
- Raise your right leg and, with your right hand, extend your right arm to the number 12.
- Then, with your arm extended, the point at the number three, then to the number six behind you. Return your arm to the number three, then again to the number twelve.
- Maintain your focus on the path ahead.
- Repeat this exercise twice more on each side.

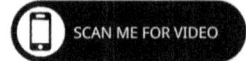

SCAN ME FOR VIDEO

This activity encourages you to consider what you're doing while improving your static balance. It also strengthens your ankle and hip muscles while increasing the range of motion of your shoulder and upper body.

Things to take care of in clock reach exercise

While exercising, breathe properly through the nose and out through the mouth. Raise your chest and take a firm stance. Look at an eye-level location on the wall. Only go as far as you are comfortable. If you can't go at 6 o'clock or it's too painful, go at 3 o'clock.

Take it to the next level.

Hold on with one finger or entirely let go of the chair. Attach a one-pound weight to your wrist or ankle for a more challenging workout.

EXERCISE 44: ALTERNATING VISION WALKS

To perform this balance exercise:

- Start at one end of the room and plant your feet hip-width apart.
- Take four or five steps forward while maintaining your head position and looking over your right shoulder.
- Take some deep breaths and turn your head to look over your left shoulder.

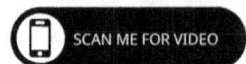

SCAN ME FOR VIDEO

- Then take another four or five steps in this position.
- Repeat the steps mentioned above five times on each shoulder.

You can hold a weight against your chest during the activity to make this exercise more challenging.

EXERCISE 45: HEAD AND THUMB SYNCHRONIZATION

After inner ear damage, a simple exercise can help the eye, inner ear, and brain re-calibrate. It's the head and thumb synchronization exercise. To perform this exercise:

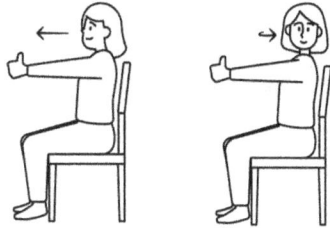

- Sit facing a blank wall and extend your thumb straight out in front of you.
- Alternatively, you can use a sticker with an "X" on a wall 3 feet or 1 meter away.
- Keep your gaze locked on your thumb or the "X" throughout this exercise.
- Turn your head to the right and then to the left.
- In a rhythmic pattern, alternate turning from left to right and back.
- It should take about 1 second to turn from left to right.
- The goal is to turn your head while keeping your gaze locked on one location. You can imagine it as your thumb or an X on the wall.
- Perform the exercise for around 1 to 2 minutes.
- Repeat this exercise 3 to 4 times a day for one to two weeks. Within one week, you should see a difference.

This activity may make you feel ill or dizzy. This does not always mean you're doing the workouts incorrectly. Do not give up. Nausea is the body's reaction to a malfunctioning inner ear. The brain will try to adapt to help recovery. Slow down the speed of your head motions and the amount you turn your head if you feel unwell for more than 30 minutes after the activity.

You may need to move your head and shoulder together if you have a stiff neck. In this scenario, using a post-it with an X on a wall is easier than using your thumb. Once you've mastered the above exercise, move on to more challenging exercises:

- Move your head faster if you can complete the exercise without feeling dizzy.
- If you can comfortably complete the exercise while sitting, try it while standing.
- Walking is an excellent way to do a workout.
- Instead of a blank wall, place your thumb or X against a busy background.
- Move your thumb slightly to the right while turning your head to the left, and vice versa.
- Try moving your head up and down instead of side to side.

Begin by sitting and gradually progress to standing or walking (with or without a busy visual background). You've done incredibly well if you can complete all of these, as often people with a healthy inner ear may struggle.

EXERCISE 46: EPLEY MANEUVER

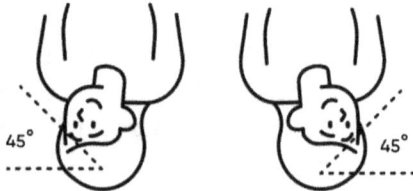

If your vertigo is coming from your left ear and side, do the following:

Take a seat at the foot of your bed. Make a 45-degree left turn with your head (not as far as your left shoulder).

- Place a pillow beneath you between your shoulders rather than under your head.
- Lie down with your head on the bed as quickly as possible (still at the 45-degree angle).

- Your pillow should be placed beneath your shoulders.
- Wait 30 seconds before continuing (for any vertigo to stop).
- Turn it halfway to the right (90 degrees).
- Wait another 30 seconds before continuing the exercise.
- Turn your body and head to the right to stare down at the ground.
- Wait another half minute.
- Sit up slowly, but stay in bed for a few minutes.

If your vertigo is coming from your right ear, follow these steps in reverse. Sit in your bed and turn your head 45 degrees to the right. Do these exercises three times each night before going to bed until you've gone 24 hours without feeling dizzy.

Are there any dangers in performing the Epley maneuver at home?

The maneuver is risk-free. Having someone accompany you through the movements at home may be beneficial. This can provide you with a peace of mind by reducing vertigo. People with health issues that limit their mobility may not be able to safely perform the Epley maneuver at home. These problems include neck or back disorders, vascular diseases, and retinal detachment. Consult your doctor to see if the home Epley maneuver is appropriate for you.

THE OUTCOME OF EPLEY MANEUVER

Most people claim that their symptoms disappear immediately after performing the maneuver. The technique may take a few attempts to work in some circumstances. For a few weeks, some people may experience moderate symptoms. There's no need to keep executing the maneuver once your symptoms have gone away. After your symptoms have subsided, your healthcare practitioner may advise you to avoid certain positions for a period. You may need to sleep propped up on two pillows to keep your neck from stretching straight.

If you do the Epley maneuver, your vertigo may disappear for weeks or even years. BPPV, on the other hand, frequently resurfaces. This could happen if another calcium stone becomes stuck in your semicircular canals. Repeat the Epley maneuver at home if your vertigo returns to see if your symptoms improve. Call your healthcare practitioner if the technique doesn't work.

EXERCISE 47: SEMONT MANEUVER

DO NOT PERFORM THIS EXERCISE WITHOUT YOUR DOCTOR OR PHYSICAL THERAPIST PRESENT

The Semont treatment is another posterior canal movement that moves debris or "ear rocks" (also known as otoconia) from the sensitive region of the ear to a less sensitive location. It takes around 15 minutes to complete the maneuver.

The Semont technique is a procedure that includes swiftly shifting the patient from one side to the other. It is comparable to the Epley technique in some perspectives because the head orientation to gravity is highly similar. In terms of the total number of positions, it is more efficient than the Epley Maneuver. Still, the biomechanics of the maneuver is a little more complicated (but not as challenging as the "Foster" maneuver).

Your physical therapist may perform the Semont technique to assist in treating your BPPV. It's a straightforward procedure that should relieve your dizziness. A physical therapist is needed to execute the Semont maneuver with you to verify that it is performed correctly and that you are kept safe throughout the treatment. You can expect the following steps during this maneuver:

- Sit on the edge of a bed or a treatment table.
- Your physical therapist will determine whether the BPPV has damaged your left or right vestibular system.
- They will move your head 45 degrees away from the affected side physically.
- After that, your physical therapist will swiftly lie you down on the side of your body that BPPV afflicts.
- Once your PT has you lying on your side, you should be staring at the ceiling.
- This pose could make you dizzy. You should keep lying on your side until your symptoms go away.
- The physical therapist will then assist you in rising to a sitting position and rapidly transferring you to your unaffected side,

keeping your head in the same position. Your gaze should now be drawn to the ground.
- This pose may again cause dizziness. Remain in the side-lying position until the dizziness subsides.
- After that, your physical therapist will help you get back into a seated posture.

You should strive to stay upright for a few hours after performing the Semont technique. The therapist may recommend that you sleep with your head propped up on a couple of pillows to keep you slightly upright overnight.

The calcium crystals of the vestibular system get repositioned using the Semont maneuver. If the treatment is successful, your vertigo symptoms should go away in a day or two. If they persist, your PT may recommend the Epley maneuver, which is already discussed.

Both the Semont and Epley movements aren't always successful in alleviating your problems. To help with BPPV treatment, your physical therapist may recommend Brandt Daroff exercises. These workouts will not reposition the calcium crystals in your vestibular system. Instead, they assist your body in becoming accustomed to and compensating for your BPPV.

Patient Instructions After Semont Maneuver

- Wait 10 minutes after completing the move before returning home. This prevents the attacks of vertigo, which occur as debris repositions itself in response to the motion.
- Do not attempt to drive yourself home.
- For the next night, sleep semi-recumbent. This entails sleeping with your head halfway between being flat and erect (at a 45-degree angle) position. A recliner chair or pillows piled on a couch are the most convenient ways to accomplish this.
- Try to keep your head erect during the day. You must not visit a hairstylist or a dentist.
- Males should lean their bodies forward to maintain their heads vertical while shaving under their chins.
- If you need to use eye drops, attempt to do so without leaning your head back. Only shampoo in the shower.

- Avoid aggravating head positions that may trigger BPPV for at least one week.
- Use two pillows while sleeping.
- Avoid sleeping on the "wrong" side of the bed.
- Don't swivel your head too far up or down.
- Avoid laying on your back in a head-extended position, especially if your head is turned to the affected side.
- Attempt to maintain as much uprightness as possible. Discontinue low-back discomfort exercises for a week.
- Avoid extreme head-forward positions, such as those found in some workouts (i.e., touching the toes)

One week after treatment, put yourself in a position that makes you dizzy most of the time. Place yourself carefully and in a safe environment where you won't fall or harm yourself. Inform your healthcare provider of your progress.

EXERCISE 48: HALF-SOMERSAULT OR FOSTER MANEUVER

DO NOT PERFORM THIS EXERCISE WITHOUT CONSULTING YOUR DOCTOR OR PHYSICAL THERAPIST FIRST

Many people who suffer from vertigo seek the help of qualified medical professionals. These experts use therapeutic techniques to clear crystals from the ear's semicircular canals. The positional episodes typically fade away within a few hours, but some can last for days. Dizzy spells frequently occur as a result of this. Others try to shift crystals away with their head movement, and DIY (do it yourself) methods are commonly used as home workouts. The half somersault maneuver is one of the few successful home exercises for vertigo.

- Kneel in the middle of a large bed or on the floor.
- Quickly tilt your head upward until you look straight up at the ceiling. This may produce dizziness for a short time.
- Next, turn your head upside down on the floor as if you're about to somersault.

- Tuck your chin in so that the back of your head, rather than the forehead, hits the floor. This position could produce a vertigo attack.
- Wait until any vertigo subsides before moving. Vertigo indicates that the particles are traveling in the correct direction. Moving the particles forward might be aided by tapping hard on the skull with your fingertips immediately behind the right ear.
- Slowly turn your head so that your right elbow is facing you.
- Try to center the right elbow in your area of vision.
- Maintain your head turned to the right throughout the motion.
- Wait for any vertigo to go away before proceeding to the following procedure.
- Raise your head to shoulder level while keeping your head turned to the right and looking at your right elbow.
- Your head should be at a 45-degree angle to the floor throughout this movement. During this portion of the operation, vertigo is common.
- Before continuing, wait for vertigo to subside or count to 15.
- Raise your head quickly to a standing position, maintaining it roughly halfway turned toward your right shoulder. There may be some additional vertigo. Sit up carefully after vertigo has subsided.
- Allow 15 minutes for rest.
- Tip your head up and down swiftly after the rest. Do not repeat the procedure if no dizziness arises.
- If you still feel dizzy after performing that movement, try it again. If you have another vertigo attack in the future, you can repeat the maneuver.

Things to take care

To allow particles to settle, wait at least 15 minutes between moves.

Sleep raised up on two or three pillows for two nights after the maneuver.

After the procedure, sleep only on your left side for a week (put a pillow behind you to keep you from rolling over in the night).

EXERCISE 49: BRANDT-DAROFF EXERCISE

DO NOT PERFORM THIS EXERCISE WITHOUT CONSULTING YOUR DOCTOR OR PHYSICAL THERAPIST FIRST

Benign Paroxysmal Positional Vertigo is treated with Brandt-Daroff exercise (BPPV).

Advantages of performing this exercises

BPPV patients can use the exercises to prevent dizzy spells. It's unclear why the exercises work; some data suggest that they help reposition the loose crystals that cause dizziness in the first place, while other evidence suggests that repeated exposure to the sensation lessens its severity.

What are the dangers or drawbacks?

Because the exercise is likely to cause dizziness, it should be done in a safe atmosphere, preferably with the help of another person. Some people have difficulty sticking with the exercise, but it has a high success rate.

Any Alternatives?

Alternative techniques, such as the Epley maneuver, can be employed to treat BPPV. Your therapist may conduct an Epley maneuver with you in the clinic. The therapist may propose Brandt-Daroff exercises for you at home because they are easier to complete without supervision.

How to Perform this Exercise

- Turn your head 45 degrees to one side while sitting comfortably sideways in the middle of the bed.
- Lay down sideways on the bed opposite to how your head is turned, keeping your head 45 degrees to one side.
- Lie down on your left side if your head is oriented to the right.
- This movement may cause dizziness or vertigo for a limited time.
- Stay in this position for 30 seconds or until the dizziness subsides, whichever comes first.
- Return to a seated position and hold it for 30 seconds.
- Turn your head 45 degrees opposite as before and repeat the procedure on the opposite side. This entails turning your head 45 degrees to one side and lying down sideways on the bed on the opposite side of where your head is turned.

- If your head is oriented to the right, lie down on your left side.
- This movement may cause a temporary feeling of dizziness once more. Stay in this position for 30 seconds or until the dizziness subsides, whichever comes first.
- Return to a seated position and hold it for 30 seconds.
- Repeat as needed, depending on your schedule.
- When you've finished your set of exercises, sit on the side of your bed until any dizziness has subsided and you feel safe standing up.

The above description is one repetition. The exercise should be done in five repetitions, three times a day for 14 days.

FOLLOW UP

After practicing any of these exercises, try not to tilt your head too far up or down for the rest of the day. If you don't feel better after a week of attempting these exercises, speak with your doctor again and ask what they recommend you do next. You could be executing the exercises incorrectly, or something else could be causing your dizziness.

CHAPTER 8
FLOOR WORK
A GROUP OF LYING DOWN EXERCISES

We have already covered standing, seated, core fitness, vertigo, and walking exercises that help improve balance. This chapter discusses the exercises that can be done while lying down on the floor.

EXERCISE 50: TRUNK ROTATION

Trunk rotation is a core-strengthening, stability, flexibility, and mobility exercise. The workout can be done in various ways, giving you the freedom to progress, challenge yourself, and do what feels right for you.

Trunk rotation is used in a variety of everyday tasks and sports participation. You complete a trunk rotation by lying on the ground, bending your knees while engaging your core, and rotating your knees from side to side.

SCAN ME FOR VIDEO

Benefits of Trunk Rotation Exercise

The trunk muscles are involved in every motion the body makes. They assist you in walking, maintaining balance, and maintaining body stability. Improving trunk mobility and strength with a rotation exercise like this can help achieve general fitness and athletic performance.

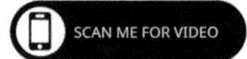

Trunk rotation is also a common rehabilitative exercise for lower back pain relief. Lower back discomfort is a prevalent complaint among older individuals. If you have back discomfort, improving trunk mobility and learning how to manage the movements of your trunk can be quite beneficial.

Trunk rotation is a simple addition to any core workout. It improves your fitness level by strengthening your trunk muscles. Trunk rotation is a movement involving the thoracic and lumbar vertebrae and the muscles surrounding them.

The trunk muscles are frequently the first to activate as you twist and move your body to help maintain stability. Exercises are essential for maintaining the optimal function of these muscles. Trunk rotation exercises can also increase trunk muscular strength, function, and mobility.

HOW TO PERFORM TRUNK ROTATION EXERCISE

Trunk rotation is a common exercise for improving the trunk muscles' strength and function. It's crucial to work at your fitness level for this activity, as it is for any exercise. The methods below will assist you in safely and correctly performing the exercise:

- Begin in a supine position (lying on your back) on an exercise mat.
- Now bend your knees, while your feet should be flat on the floor.
- Keep a firm grip on the floor with your shoulders and upper chest.
- Extend your arms and press them into the floor to help you stay balanced during the activity.
- Now slowly and deliberately rotate your knees to one side, working within your range of motion. Your feet will shift but should stay on the ground.
- Hold this position for a few seconds.
- To transfer your legs to the opposite side, engage/tighten your core muscles.
- Hold for a few more seconds.
- Throughout the activity, stay concentrated and breathe regularly.
- Repeat the exercise for a certain number of repetitions on each side

Common Mistakes During Trunk Rotation Exercise

Although trunk rotation appears to be a simple bodyweight exercise, it requires careful attention to form and technique. The following are some common blunders to avoid when doing this activity.

Working Beyond Your Fitness Level

Trunk rotation requires a certain fitness level and meticulous attention to precision, like any other workout. The activity should provide a challenging workout without overworking the muscles.

Because it's a bodyweight workout, some people overdo it, inflicting more harm than good. Begin slowly and gradually increase your strength and spinal mobility over time.

Failure to Engage the Core

The workout requires tightening your abdominal core muscles throughout the trunk rotation movement. The exercise is incorrectly performed if you merely move your legs back and forth without engaging your core muscles.

It may not feel comfortable on your low back if you aren't utilizing the proper muscles. To ease any discomfort, concentrate on activating your core.

Incorrect Range of Motion

Trunk rotation is a tiny, slow, and controlled movement. The goal isn't to see if you can touch each side of the floor with your knees. Rather than performing a significant movement, the idea is to control the motion. Work within a suitable range of motion for a correctly executed and effective workout.

Precautions and Safety

Trunk rotation has been proven to help enhance spinal mobility, flexibility, and core strength. The following pointers can help you avoid injury and maintain appropriate form during the movement:

- Keep your body attentive throughout the exercise to ensure good form and technique.

- Engage your core during the workout to efficiently execute the action without risking low-back discomfort or injury. Imagine your navel being sucked into your spine.
- Slowly and steadily do the exercise. Perform ten reps on each side.
- Concentrate on controlling the motion rather than increasing it. Use a lower range of motion for stronger trunk muscles.
- Perform the exercise according to your fitness level and range of motion in your spine.
- Use the right exercise progression concepts (add challenges only when you have mastered the basic movement).
- You should stop if you suffer pain or discomfort that doesn't seem right throughout the workout.

EXERCISE 51: STRAIGHT LEG RAISES TO THE BACK

Leg workout activities help strengthen the lower body, promoting balance and flexibility; as a result, functional independence and confidence rise.

Make sure your low back is pressed into the floor when your straight leg rises. This aligns with your spine, which improves your safety and comfort.

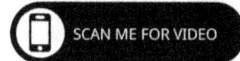

SCAN ME FOR VIDEO

This leg training exercise is excellent because:

- Increases leg and hip strength and low back and pelvic stability.
- It aims to get you to think about what you're doing.
- Strengthens your quadriceps and hip flexors.
- Makes your abdominal muscles stronger.
- Allows you to walk more easily by allowing you to advance your leg.
- Here is how you can do straight leg raises:
- Lie down on your back with one knee bent and the other straight; your toes pointed to the ceiling.
- Raise your straightened leg to the same level as the bent knee on the other side.
- Return to the starting position and repeat ten times more with each leg.

Breathing

During the upward movement phase, inhale. During the downward movement phase, exhale.

Tips for a better experience with this exercise

· Place your palms down to gain greater support.

· During the lifting portion, exhale.

· Do not lift one knee higher than the other.

· Take it to the next level.

· Place a 2 to 5-pound weight on your ankle for this leg workout.

· Stay in the raised position for 10 seconds.

EXERCISE 52: BRIDGES

If you find yourself sitting a lot, the bridge exercise, also known as the glute bridge, might help keep your lower body active.

This exercise engages the posterior chain (the muscles on the back of your body). It is a powerful glute activation exercise commonly used in lower body training.

SCAN ME FOR VIDEO

Glute bridges and other glute-focused exercises can be done at any time of the day – try them first thing in the morning, during lunch, or at the end of the day. Activating the correct muscles during a workout might be difficult if you have tight hips or under-active glutes. Completing regular activation exercises can help you strengthen your glutes appropriately.

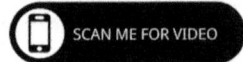

What is a bridge exercise?

The gluteus (butt) muscles – the gluteus maximus, medius, and minimus — and the hamstrings, which make up the posterior thigh, are isolated and strengthened with a bridge exercise.

The exercise is done by lying on your back with your knees bent. You will keep your feet level on the ground, and your butt at a comfortable distance. The glute bridge is a no-equipment exercise that may be performed while lying on a fitness or yoga mat or a towel.

A glute bridge is easy enough to do at any age or fitness level, yet it's difficult enough that you'll notice the results long after you've finished your workout.

You can combine the glute bridge with other exercises to achieve a full-body workout or use it as part of your warm-up.

How to perform the Bridges Exercise?

Instead of lifting your hips high, focus on engaging your glutes, which can create lower back pain and damage when you stretch through the lumbar spine.

Keep your core and glutes tight, and press through your heels to raise your hips with each repetition. A resistance band wrapped across your knees might assist you in keeping your knees pulled out and activating your glutes.

- Begin on a yoga mat by lying flat on your back.
- Bend your knees and place your feet firmly on the mat, making sure they are hip-width apart and your spine is neutral.
- Allow your arms to rest on the carpet by your sides. This is where you'll begin.
- Press your heels into the mat, tighten your glutes, and lift your pelvis off the floor. Do it until your body is straight from the chin to the knee, with your shoulders on the carpet.
- Inhale.
- Return to the beginning posture by lowering your pelvis.
- Repeat the moves a few times.

Benefits of Bridge Exercise

The bridge exercise is ideal for an at-home workout because it requires minimal equipment and little room. It's a wonderful exercise for hip mobility and lower back strength, and because it's low-impact, it's ideal for anyone with knee or hip problems.

Because the glutes are one of the largest muscular groups in the body, training them requires a lot of energy. As a result, the glute bridge is a beneficial workout for women who want to shed weight or develop power.

These muscles are also quite important because you utilize them every day for walking, carrying a big laundry basket, and taking out the trash! The glute bridge can also help enhance core stability and lower back and hip strength, improving your balance and posture.

EXERCISE 53: CLAM SHELLS

It appears too good to be true. How can a single exercise help with so many different aches and pains? The explanation is that it performs a fantastic job targeting the glute muscles, especially the gluteus medius.

It would help if you had solid and coordinated glute muscles to anchor your pelvis, manage hip joint movement, and maintain excellent knee alignment. When standing or moving on one leg, this is especially true. The exercise which provides all these benefits is clamshells.

The exercise strengthens the glute muscles, particularly the gluteus medius muscles on the sides of the hips, aiding pelvic support and stability and improving standing balance.

How to perform Clam Shells Exercise?

To complete this activity, follow these steps:

- Lie on your side with your knees bowed and stacked on top of one another.
- Your lower arm supports your head while your other arm focuses on your pelvis.
- Slightly roll forward so that your top hand is in front of your bottom hip bone (this ensures we target the glutes and not hip flexors)
- Slightly tighten the abdominal muscles (30 percent of max)
- Lift your top knee away from your bottom knee, maintaining your ankles as close together as possible without displacing your pelvis.
- Rest for a minute, then repeat for three sets of ten repetitions.

- Return to your starting place and repeat the process.
- Turn over and repeat on the other side!

Make this exercise more challenging.

Follow these instructions to take this activity to the next level:

- Place a resistance band around your thighs above your knees and lie on your side with your knees bent and knees and ankles stacked.
- Lift your knee toward the ceiling while keeping your ankles together. Allowing your body or hips to roll backward is not a good idea.
- Hold for three seconds before bringing your knees together again.
- Repeat for a total of 10 reps, then swap sides.
- Rest, then repeat on each side for a total of three sets of ten repetitions.

EXERCISE 54: LEG RAISES

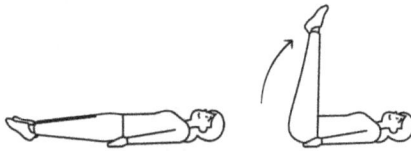

Integrate leg raises in your strength-training program if you're searching for a basic ab workout to help you create a strong core.

What exactly is Leg Raises Exercise?

Leg raises, also known as straight leg raises or lying leg raises, are bodyweight workouts that target the lower abdomen muscles. When done correctly, leg lifts train muscle groups all over your body, including the rectus abdominis, hip flexor muscles, hamstrings, and lower back muscles. Try adding ankle weights or attempting the hanging leg raise for a more advanced form.

Leg Raises: How to Do Them Right?

If you are a beginner, do the Leg lifts in 2 to 3 sets of 10 to 15 reps to begin. Your ability to maintain appropriate technique throughout the whole range of motion should determine the number of sets and repetitions you do.

- Keep your legs straight and feet together while lying down on an exercise mat.
- Place your arms at your sides, palms down, behind your glutes, or at your sides with palms facing down.
- Involve your abdominal muscles.
- Lift your legs a few inches off the ground and point your toes away from your body while maintaining straight legs.
- Throughout the action, keep your chin tucked as if you were holding an egg beneath your chin.
- Your ribs should be down, and your pelvis should be tucked in. This is the beginning point for all repetitions.
- Raise your legs until your knees are exactly above your hips ensure your glutes are slightly elevated off the ground while maintaining alignment.
- Make a 90-degree angle with your legs and upper torso.
- At the end of the movement, take a slight pause.
- Maintaining your core engaged and your upper body in contact with the workout mat, slowly drop your legs until they are just over the ground.
- At the bottom of the movement, come to a complete stop.
- Repeat until you've reached the desired number of repetitions.

Leg Raises Variations

It's simple to make this workout fun and challenging by using a variety of leg lift variations. A common form of this technique for novices is to lie down on your back, lift your feet off the ground, and bend your knees to a 90-degree angle. This position will allow no gaps between your back and the floor to form. Slowly lower and tap one heel to the floor at a time, alternating the legs while holding both legs above the ground. You can also alter the practice by slowing down the tempo to regulate the action better.

You can also add the resistance to increase the intensity. Place a medicine ball between your legs at the ankles and steadily lower and raise the weight while squeezing it. Make sure your back is firmly on the floor and there are no gaps. Your range of motion and the depth your legs can reach while maintaining proper form may be limited due to the increased resistance.

Another option is to make a 'T' shape with your hands by stretching them to the side. The abdominal muscles are emphasized more as a result of this. Leg lifts can also be done seated on an elevated surface with your hands behind your back, raising your torso and compressing your abdominal muscles.

EXERCISE 55: LYING SIDE HIP RAISE

The lying side hip raise is a great body-weight exercise that engages various muscles. The primary target muscles are the obliques essential for moving the spine and stabilizing the pelvic and lower back, but the traps and shoulders are also targeted. The exercise is comparable to a plank but with repetitions; thus, this core stabilization action benefits the entire core.

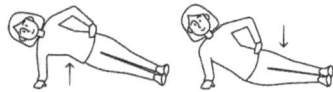

However, the lying side hip lift is a simple and effective workout that requires no equipment other than a soft surface. As a result, integrate this exercise into your ab program for even better core development.

How to do this exercise?

- Lie on one side of a yoga mat, lengthwise, with your legs piled on top.
- Place your forearm firmly on the floor, with your elbow squarely below your shoulder and your forearm parallel to (in line with) the mat's short edge.
- Bend both knees to a 90-degree angle, keeping your legs together so your shins are behind you. This is where you'll begin.
- To engage your core, gently draw your ribs to your hips.
- Using your obliques to gently lift your hips off the mat while keeping your feet together, ensure that your body is straight from head to knee.
- At the same time, raise your upper knee towards the ceiling with your glutes. It ensures that the gap between your waist and the floor is maintained.
- As you do this, your glutes should feel tense.

- Return to the beginning posture by lowering your knees and hips.
- On each side, repeat for the appropriate number of repetitions.

Because this workout involves coordination and strength, it's critical to maintain a regular breathing pattern.

Things to Consider During Lying Side Hip Raises

Maintain a straight posture with your legs and body.

Bend your knees and support your lower body on the side of your knee instead of the side of your foot to make the lying side hip lift exercise simpler.

Holding a weight on your hip will make the exercise more challenging.

Allowing your neck to rest on your shoulder is not a good idea. By extending your shoulder, you may maintain a distance between the two.

The side hip raise is also known as the side plank hip drop, side bridge hip raise, and hip-up.

BONUS* EXERCISE 56: KNEE TO CHEST POSE EXERCISE

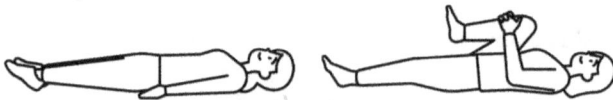

You are not alone if you ever feel like you miss the point when attempting a lower back stretch, even though you know specific muscles are incredibly tight and make every effort to release them. For many of us, stretching the hip, neck, calf, and other muscles is a simple process.

But what about the back muscles? Not at all. These can become difficult to reach if they grow too tight. Finding the sweet spot for stretchiness in the lower back muscles can be challenging if you don't choose the correct exercise for the job.

To improve back flexibility, you can conduct a continuous toe touch. Yes, you're rounding your back, which theoretically stretches those muscles, but the movement of toe contact occurs predominantly at the hip joints. Back rounding is often a consequence of this and is also not incredibly safe.

The knees-to-chest stretch comes in handy here. It feels fantastic, but it's also an excellent technique to re-establish flexibility in your lower back muscles after gardening, housekeeping, or a day at the computer.

However, the knees-to-chest stretch benefits more than just releasing lower back muscles. The knees-to-chest stretch, a range of motion exercise that develops joint flexibility, may help alleviate stiffness associated with spinal arthritis and spinal stenosis. Range of motion exercises can help persons with osteoarthritis lubricate their joints, enhance blood flow, and provide nutrients to the affected area. This exercise strengthens your hip flexors and extensors at the same time. Because it helps expand the lower back, hips, and thighs, it's a popular yoga move for seniors. It also promotes proper blood circulation in the hip area.

How to Perform Knee to Chest Exercise?

- Lie down on your back. Keep your knees bent and feet flat on the floor.
- Raise one bent knee to the point where you can hold your lower leg with both hands. Interlace your fingers just below the knee.
- Bring one leg up first, then the other, if you're doing the two-legged version. Because taking both up requires a lot of abdominal power, it's probably safest to start with one and then immediately follow with the other, especially for people with weak backs.
- As you did with the single-legged version, interlace your fingers or clasp your wrists between the lower thighs below the knees if you're doing both legs simultaneously.
- Gently bring your bent knee or knees toward your trunk using your hands.
- While pulling, try to relax your legs, pelvis, and low back as much as possible. The knees-to-chest position reaches the lower back muscles more effectively when utilized passively.
- Hold this position for a few seconds.
- Bring your leg back to the floor.
- Repeat on the opposite side.
- Stretch for 10 to 15 minutes, once or twice a day, or as needed.

Stretching in a Chain

Knees-to-chest should be done as a passive stretch with the legs and hips as relaxed as possible. This may help you attain exceptional spinal flexion by allowing the natural chain reaction from the thigh to the hip to the low back.

To put it another way, the bottom of your pelvis should slightly elevate when you pull your thigh to your chest. Most likely, the pulling will continue up your spine until it reaches your lumbar spine. If you're having trouble getting that lift in your lower pelvis, try placing a small towel or folded blanket beneath the base of your tailbone to assist you in getting started.

If you are finding this book useful, please take 60 seconds to leave a review so others can take advantage of these cool concepts, as reviews help others find what they need. Thank you so much for your attention and participation!
https://www.amazon.com/review/create-review?&asin=B0C2B2JQ9P

Customer reviews
★★★★☆ 4.5 out of 5
25 global ratings

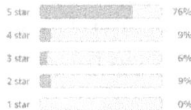

5 star	76%
4 star	9%
3 star	6%
2 star	9%
1 star	0%

⌄ How customer reviews and ratings work

Review this product
Share your thoughts with other customers

Write a customer review

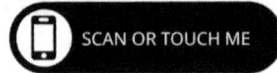

SCAN OR TOUCH ME

CHAPTER 9
DISEASES THAT CAUSE BALANCE ISSUES IN SENIORS

T his chapter discusses the common diseases that occur in old age and their effects on balance. We will also discuss the preventive measures and exercises to regain the lost balance.

PARKINSON'S DISEASE

Parkinson's disease is a degenerative brain condition affecting people as they age. It damages the portions of the brain. The disease is commonly known for causing delayed movements, tremors, and balance issues. Unknown factors cause most cases; however, some are hereditary. Although the illness is not curable, there are numerous treatment options available.

PARKINSONISM AND BALANCE ISSUES

Parkinson's disease (PD) can alter a person's walking style. Movement It's more challenging to take typical steps when you have symptoms like stiff muscles, rigidity, and delayed movement. In reality, short, shuffling steps are a common symptom for those with mid-stage to advanced PD, as is freezing or the sensation that your feet are stuck to the floor.

These changes are stressful enough on their own. However, when Parkinson's disease affects balance, they become dangerous, placing patients with PD at risk of falling. The good news is that patients with PD can improve their balance with exercise and physical treatment.

CAUSES OF FALLS IN PATIENTS WITH PARKINSON'S DISEASE

Identifying the reason or causes of falls is essential in preventing them. Although most individuals with Parkinson's disease may fall for the same core reasons, several aspects must be considered.

One of the four cardinal symptoms of Parkinson's disease is postural instability (along with rest tremors, bradykinesia or slowness of movements, and rigidity or stiffness). The inability to regain balance after being thrown off balance is known as postural instability. It's usually tested in the doctor's office when the neurologist pulls your shoulders backward to check if you can keep yourself from falling. If a person with PD with postural instability is jostled, they may fall. This symptom does not usually appear early in the disease, although it appears as it develops.

Freezing of Gait

This is an aberrant gait pattern that can occur with Parkinson's disease (as well as other parkinsonian disorders). You have unexpected, brief, and transitory episodes in which you cannot move your feet forward despite your best efforts. In some ways, you're trapped. As a result, the feet take on the typical appearance of quick-stepping movements in position. While the feet remain in position, the torso continues to move forward, resulting in common falls in the context of gait freezing.

Festinating Gait

Festinating gait is another irregular walking pattern that can arise in persons with Parkinson's disease. In this gait, the person takes small, quick steps that get smaller and quicker until they appear to be running. The person may not be able to stop walking in this pattern and may end up hitting walls to come to a halt. Falling is a risk of festination.

Dyskinesias

Dyskinesias are other involuntary movements that some people experience as a side effect of taking Levodopa, a type of medicine used to treat

Parkinson's. Dyskinesias can throw a person off balance and cause falls if the unexpected movements are severe.

Visuospatial Impairment

Visuospatial impairment is one of the most common cognitive problems that patients with PD face. The incapacity to navigate in three dimensions is caused by deficits in this cognitive domain. A person may struggle to navigate around obstructions in a room or back up to sit in a chair. Falls can occur as a result of these difficulties.

Orthostatic Hypotension

Orthostatic hypotension — Your blood pressure lowers when you change your head position. This is a common non-motor symptom of Parkinson's disease. This can cause dizziness and even passing out, which a bystander may misinterpret as a fall.

PREVENTION OF FALLS

Knowing which causes contribute to falls is critical because each cause is treated differently.

Increases in PD medicines may help with postural instability in Parkinson's patients.

Increasing the medication dose might sometimes help alleviate gait freeze and festination.

Adjusting the dose of medicines or starting amantadine can help with bothersome dyskinesias.

Orthostatic hypotension can be treated with various techniques, including increased fluid intake, dietary salt, and compression stockings. Medications to raise blood pressure can also be explored if necessary.

EXERCISES TO IMPROVE BALANCE IN PARKINSONISM

Balance exercises alone, balance exercises mixed with strengthening exercises, cueing, treadmill gait training, tai chi, and functional training have all enhanced balance control in people with Parkinson's disease.

Following exercises can help Parkinson's patients regain their lost balance. These exercises have already been discussed in the book.

- Static standing balance
- Tandem standing
- Tandem walk
- Single leg stand
- Lateral weight shift
- Sidestepping
- Backward walking
- Zig zag walking

ALZHEIMER'S DISEASE

Alzheimer's is the most common form of dementia. It's a progressive condition that starts with mild memory loss and progresses to losing the ability to converse and respond to the environment. The disease affects the regions of the brain involved in thought, memory, and behavior. It can significantly impact a person's capacity to carry out daily tasks.

One of the first signs of Alzheimer's disease is forgetting recent events or talks. As the condition progresses, a person with Alzheimer's disease will have severe memory loss and lose the ability to do daily tasks.

Medications can temporarily improve or minimize the severity of symptoms. These medications can sometimes help people with Alzheimer's disease maintain their independence while maximizing their function. A wide range of programs and services are available to people with Alzheimer's disease and their caregivers.

THE LINK BETWEEN THE MIND AND THE BODY

Though the cause of Alzheimer's disease is unknown, scientists believe that the symptoms are caused by an accumulation of toxic proteins called amyloid and tau in the brain. Tangles and plaques are large masses formed by the collection of these proteins. They obstruct regular brain activity and cause the death of healthy cells.

The damage usually begins in the memory-forming region of the brain. Early-stage Alzheimer's disease patients sometimes have problems recalling things. Plaques and clusters appear in the brain areas that control physiological activities as the disease progresses.

Walking, eating, going to the restroom, and talking grow more complex. The effects vary from person to person as the condition progresses.

PHYSICAL CHANGES

Everyone is different regarding which symptoms they experience and when they arise. Before significant memory loss, some persons experience physical issues.

The following are some of the changes you may notice:

- Loss of coordination or balance
- Muscle spasms
- Walking with shuffled or dragging feet
- Standing or sitting up in a chair is difficult.
- Muscle weakness and exhaustion
- Sleep disorders
- Problems managing your bladder or bowels.
- Uncontrollable twitches and seizures

BALANCE ISSUES IN ALZHEIMER'S DISEASE

The most prevalent side symptoms of Alzheimer's disease and related dementias are memory problems and difficulty thinking. Still, the loss of balance is a frightening issue that caregivers should be aware of, especially as the condition progresses.

Losing balance while standing or walking can suggest an increased risk of Alzheimer's disease in its early stages, even before other dementia symptoms appear. It could also indicate that your loved one has dementia other than Alzheimer's, such as vascular dementia.

The cerebellum, which is positioned near the back base of the skull, is the region of the brain that controls body motions. Balance is likely to be affected by diseases that affect the cerebellum, and certain varieties of dementia match the bill. Vascular dementia, for example, differs from Alzheimer's disease in that it is caused by a loss of blood supply to the cerebellum, which results in a shortage of oxygen. (Multi-infarct dementia is another name for Vascular dementia). Before people develop problems with thinking and memory, some persons with vascular dementia will have vertigo (the sensation of moving when standing motionless).

There is also a type of Alzheimer's disease known as "posterior cortical atrophy," which affects balance by affecting the cerebellum. People with posterior cortical atrophy may lose their feeling of which direction is up, be more prone to dizziness, and lean to one side more frequently.

Balance loss is frequent in persons with Alzheimer's disease, especially in the later stages. Late-stage Alzheimer's patients often have difficulty seeing, interpreting information about the physical environment, and walking. These difficulties result from brain cells degenerating and deterioration of neuronal connectivity throughout the body. All of these have an impact on the equilibrium. A standard adjustment is changing one's "gait," or walking style, to shuffle their feet instead of lifting them with each stride. Walking this way is more complex, and you're more likely to lose your balance and fall. Workouts like Tai Chi, stationary cycling, and leg lifts are beneficial.

HOW TO IMPROVE BALANCE IN ALZHEIMER'S DISEASE?

People with dementia benefit from regular exercise because it improves their balance and lowers their reliance on others.

Exercise, in general, can help seniors maintain their flexibility and strength. This is necessary for reducing the risk of falling. Strength training, stretching, and stamina-building exercises are the most effective.

Here are a few senior-friendly forms of exercise to try with your loved one:

Restorative Yoga

Yoga strengthens the core and improves overall flexibility. While many people connect yoga with complex floor-based techniques, there are alternative options. For people with mobility issues, chair yoga can be beneficial and safer.

Walking

Most people know that walking is benefits heart health, but it does more. It also improves bone density and relieves stress. Walking is an excellent activity for persons with dementia because of the mind-body link.

Tai Chi

This ancient Chinese practice is a wonderful choice for persons with dementia because of its slow, consistent movements. It will help you improve your balance, stamina, and core strength and help you sleep better. People with Alzheimer's and dementia frequently have difficulty falling asleep.

Lightweight training

An older adult's core strength can be improved by using small hand weights or resistance bands. According to research, repetition is the key to building a more substantial body during retirement.

Working with an occupational therapist is a final suggestion. These medical specialists can figure out how to work with a dementia patient's physical limitations. An occupational therapist can help an older adult overcome difficulties by reaching up or kneeling to get items from a shelf.

DIABETIC NEUROPATHY

Diabetes can cause nerve damage. The damage is called neuropathy and can be painful.

Diabetic neuropathy can manifest itself in various ways, all of which appear to be linked to blood sugar levels that have been elevated for an extended time. Work with your doctor to keep your blood sugar under control to avoid it.

TYPES OF DIABETIC NEUROPATHY

Peripheral, autonomic, proximal, and focal neuropathy are the four types of diabetes-related neuropathy. Peripheral neuropathy is the type that causes balance issues in seniors.

Peripheral Neuropathy

Peripheral neuropathy is a diabetic neuropathy that affects the feet and legs. Arms, abdomen, and back are also affected in rare circumstances.

The symptoms include:

1. Tingling
2. Feelings of numbness (which may become permanent)
3. Burning sensation
4. Pain

When your blood sugar is under control, your early symptoms usually improve. There are drugs available to help alleviate the pain.

BALANCE ISSUES IN DIABETIC NEUROPATHY

Diabetic peripheral neuropathy might cause you to walk with an unsteady stride or perhaps lose your balance. This is generally made more accessible by wearing orthopedic shoes.

A loss of coordination characterizes diabetic peripheral neuropathy. Muscle weakness frequently affects the ankle, which might alter your walk. Loss of balance can also be caused by numbness in the feet.

The presence and severity of diabetic peripheral neuropathy have been linked with postural instability (DPN). People with peripheral diabetic neuropathy have been shown to sway more than people of similar age and health when silently standing with their eyes open. People with diabetic neuropathy have the most significant loss of postural stability when their eyes are closed.

Furthermore, frequent falls have been linked to a loss of vibration sensation and a loss of pressure sensitivity. Older persons with diabetes walk slower and have more stride variability due to diminished cognitive feedback during walking; these characteristics increase the risk of falling. Similarly, there are strong links between diabetic retinopathy, diabetes duration, and the risk of falling.

Adults over 70 years of age with diabetes have been reported to have a higher risk of incurring more serious injuries following a fall as well as having a higher risk of falling. Despite having similar bone mineral densities, seniors with diabetes have a greater risk of fractures than those without diabetes.

This deterioration in bone quality could be linked to greater levels of advanced glycation end products in the bones. Bone fractures increase by 64 percent in people with diabetes compared to healthy people.

BALANCE EXERCISES FOR DIABETIC NEUROPATHY

Peripheral neuropathy can cause stiffness and weakness in your muscles and joints. Balance training may aid in the development of strength and the reduction of tension. Falling is also less likely when one's balance is improved. Leg and calf raises are fundamental balancing exercises.

Other exercises that can improve balance in diabetic neuropathy include:

- Side leg raise
- Calf raises
- Calf stretch
- Seated hamstring stretch

These exercises have already been discussed in detail. You can follow the instructions and regain your lost balance.

OSTEOARTHRITIS

Osteoarthritis is a common disease that affects any joint in the body. The joints that carry most of our weight, such as the knees and feet, are most prone. Joints that we frequently use in our daily lives, such as the joints in our hands, are commonly affected.

A healthy joint has a coating of tough, smooth, and slippery cartilage covering the surface of the bones, allowing them to move freely against each other. As a joint develops osteoarthritis, part of the cartilage thins, and the surface gets rougher. This means that the joint isn't moving as freely as it should.

All tissues within the joint become more active than usual as the body strives to heal the harm produced by worn or injured cartilage. Although the repair processes change the joint structure, they usually allow it to function correctly and without pain or stiffness. Even if we aren't aware of it, almost all of us will get osteoarthritis in some of our joints.

However, the repair processes aren't always successful, and alterations in the joint structure might result in or contribute to symptoms like pain, swelling, or difficulty moving the joint normally.

SYMPTOMS

The most common symptoms of osteoarthritis are pain and stiffness in the affected joints. The discomfort is usually worse when you move the joint or near the end of a long day. Your joints may feel stiff after rest, but this usually passes once you resume moving. Changes in symptoms might occur for no apparent reason. You can also find that your symptoms change depending on what you're doing.

Swelling of the afflicted joint is possible. The swelling could be caused by:

Extra bone growth that causes the skin to become stiff and knobbly, especially finger joints.

Due to a thickening of the joint lining and excess fluid inside the joint capsule, the joint becomes mushy.

When you move the joint, it may not move as freely or as far as it should, making grating or crackling sounds. Crepitus is the medical term for this.

The muscles around the joint may appear thin or wasted at times. Because your muscles have deteriorated or the joint structure has grown less stable, the joint may sometimes give way.

BALANCE ISSUES IN OSTEOARTHRITIS

Balance can be affected in people with osteoarthritis due to decreased joint proprioception caused by foot deformities and arthritis in the lower extremities, muscular weakness, joint mobility limitations, or central nervous system damage. Impaired balance and muscle weakness are two major risk factors for falls in patients with osteoarthritis.

In patients with bilateral knee osteoarthritis, balance (static and dynamic) in either foot position is compromised. The impairment appears to be more pronounced in moderate osteoarthritis than in mild osteoarthritis. The impaired balance in patients is also associated with an increased chance of falling.

IMPROVE BALANCE IN OSTEOARTHRITIS

Since osteoarthritis is the disease of joints, exercises are recommended to improve balance and add strength, flexibility, and posture.

Do these exercises if you are having balance issues due to osteoarthritis.

Single-Leg Stand

To perform this exercise:

Stand on one leg near a counter to catch yourself.

Lift one leg off the ground for 10 seconds.

Do the same on the opposite leg.

Work up to one minute on each leg.

Tandem stand

Put one foot in front of the other, with the toes of the back foot touching the front foot's heel.

Switch sides after 10 seconds of holding.

Work up to one minute on each leg.

Chair Stand

As the name says, this exercise involves standing up from a chair without using your hands. Work your way up to 10 repetitions.

STROKE

A stroke, also known as a brain attack, occurs when blood flow to the brain is interrupted. It's a life-or-death situation.

The brain requires a steady supply of oxygen and nutrients to function correctly. Even if the blood flow is interrupted for a brief period, this can cause issues. Brain cells begin to die without blood or oxygen after only a few minutes.

Brain function is lost when brain cells die. Possibly, you won't be able to do tasks that require that section of your brain. A stroke, for example, may impair your ability to:

- Move
- Speak
- Eat
- Consider and recall
- Control bowel and bladder
- Keep your emotions under check.
- Other critical physiological functions that are under your control

ANYONE, AT ANY TIME, CAN HAVE A STROKE.

EFFECTS OF STROKE ON BALANCE

A stroke frequently produces weakness on one side of the body, making it difficult to maintain balance. You may find it challenging to sit up safely or stand in the worst-case scenario. You might be able to walk, but you can't get your toes to rise quickly enough to keep them from sticking on the ground when you step.

How does stroke affect balance?

Different body elements, such as the brain, eyes, and limbs, must work together to achieve proper balance. Your balancing system and how the parts work together can be affected after a stroke. Your body can usually overcome minor issues, but if they get more serious, your system will be unable to function correctly, and you will likely feel unstable.

Weakness on one side of the body

A stroke frequently produces weakness on one side of the body, making it difficult to maintain balance. You may find it challenging to sit up safely or stand in the worst-case scenario. You may be able to walk, but you cannot lift your toes quickly enough to prevent them from sticking on the ground when you step. This is referred to as foot drop, and it might make you feel shaky or increase your chances of tripping. Alternatively, you may discover that you have less energy, causing you to fatigue quickly and become shaky.

Sensitivity loss

The lack of sensation in your affected side, particularly your legs, is the second major factor influencing balance. It's tough to know how to move if you can't feel where your leg and foot are, especially when your foot is safely on the ground. You'll instantly compensate for the lack of feeling with your vision, which requires a lot of concentration and is exhausting. You may also be less conscious of your surroundings as a result. All of this raises your chances of slipping, tripping, and falling.

EXERCISES TO REGAIN THE LOST BALANCE AFTER A STROKE

There are specific muscle areas that you should train to improve your full-body coordination after a stroke. Furthermore, each patient will benefit from different treatment options because each stroke is unique. Experimenting with different ways until you find one that works best for you is often beneficial.

Here are some of the most effective exercises for regaining balance after a stroke:

Beginner Level Exercises

Basic balance exercises may appear simple at first, but they require solid neural connections to accomplish correctly. Start with these simple activities. The repeated movements will help to form mental connections that will aid in the restoration of balance. Always grasp onto something to keep from falling during these beginner-level activities.

1. Heel Raises (Holding On)

Three sets of ten repetitions in each

Look for a strong chair or counter to lean on for support. Raise yourself onto your tiptoes while hanging on to the chair or counter. Keep your knees straight and your upper body tall. Slowly lower yourself to the floor and repeat.

2. Side Stepping (Holding On)

Three sets of 10 reps each (1 rep Equals each foot)

Intermediate Level Exercises

The intermediate-level exercises use the same concepts as the basic exercises, but they don't require holding anything in your hands. You should be able to complete the basic level exercises without help after some practice.

However, always have a counter or chair close to your grip if you start to lose your balance.

3. Heel Raises (Not Holding On)

Three sets of ten repetitions each

Stand with your arms at your sides and your feet flat on the floor. Raise yourself to your tiptoes, maintaining a straight upper body and knees. Lower the weight gradually and repeat.

4. Side Stepping

3 x 10 reps (1 rep Equals each foot)

Perform the side step by crossing your legs and moving sideways in a straight line without holding on to anything. To avoid falling, take it slowly and be prepared to grip something if you lose your balance.

5. Heel-to-Toe Walking

A total of 20 steps (10 for each foot)

Walk forward, placing the heel of one foot directly in front of the toe of the other as you walk, using the straight tape line for sidestepping. Continue until the end of the tape, turn, and begin again from the beginning.

ADVANCED LEVEL EXERCISES TO REGAIN BALANCE AFTER STROKE

Do not stop exercising once you notice an improvement in your balance. Those connections are still being formed. Now it's time to progress to more challenging exercises.

7. Single Leg Standing

Three sets of five repetitions

Place both of your feet flat on the ground. Slowly raise one leg until the other leg is balanced. Hold for a count of ten, then slowly lower it. Rep with the other leg.

8. Backwards Walking

A total of 20 steps

Slowly walk backward into a room that is free of impediments. To avoid falling, try not to look where you're going and instead rely on your sense of balance and slow movements. Perform this exercise using something nearby to grab onto at first, such as a wall or a counter, until you acquire confidence in your abilities.

CHAPTER 10
THE PLAN
A WEEKLY WORKOUT ROUTINE

We have discussed almost all the exercises that can be helpful to improve your balance in old age. Now is the time to make a weekly schedule and include the exercises from basic to advanced levels. Follow this routine, and you will note considerable improvement in your equilibrium and balance.

Some Points to Note About Weekly Routine

Each week will require three days of exercise.

Do these exercises on Monday, Wednesday, and Friday, but you can customize workout days according to your schedule and feasibility.

Week 1: Standing Strong, Core Fitness, Verti-Go Away

Day 1 Routine

- Seated Knee to Chest Two sets / six reps / 30-second rest between sets
- Overhead Side Stretch Two sets / eight reps / 30-second rest between sets
- Shoulder Stretch Two sets / eight reps / 30-second rest between sets
- Standing Toe Taps Two sets / ten reps (5 each side) / 30-second rest
- Side Bends Two sets / ten reps (5 each side) / 30-second rest

- Head Rotation Two sets / ten reps (5 each side) / 30-second rest

Day 2 Routine

- Hamstring Stretch. Two sets / six reps / 30 seconds rest after each set
- Soleus Stretch Two sets / four reps / 30 seconds rest
- Standing Quad Stretch Two sets / eight reps / 30 seconds rest
- Tandem Stance 2 Sets / 30 seconds each (alternate feet) / 30 sec rest
- Tightrope Walk Two sets / 20 to 30 steps each / 30 seconds rest
- Clock Reach 2 sets / left arm & right arm / 30 seconds rest

Day 3 Routine

- Shoulder Stretch Two sets / eight reps / 30-second rest between sets
- Seated Knee to Chest Two sets / six reps / 30-second rest between sets
- Triceps Stretch Two sets / eight reps / 30-second rest between sets
- Squats Two sets / eight squats / 30 seconds rest
- Plank Two sets / 10-second plank / 30 seconds rest
- Head and Thumb Sync Two sets / ten reps each arm / 30 seconds rest

Week 2: Watch Your Step, Floor Work, Verti-Go Away

Day 1 Routine

- Shoulder Stretch Two sets / eight reps / 30-second rest between sets
- Soleus Stretch Two sets / four reps / 30-second rest between sets
- Standing Quad Stretch Two sets / eight reps / 30 seconds rest
- Walking on spot Three sets / Walk for 20 seconds / 30 seconds rest
- Bridges Two sets / Ten reps / 30 seconds rest
- Clock Reach Two sets / left arm & right arm / 30 seconds rest

Day 2 Routine

- Standing Quad Stretch Two sets / eight reps / 30-second rest between sets
- Seated Knee to Chest Two sets / six reps / 30-second rest between sets
- Overhead Side Stretch Two sets / eight reps / 30 seconds rest
- Backward Steps Three sets / 10 steps / 30 seconds rest
- Leg Raises Two sets / Eight reps / 30 seconds rest
- Epley Manuever Two sets / Three reps each side / 30 seconds rest

Day 3 Routine

- Standing Quad Stretch Two sets / eight reps / 30-second rest between sets
- Seated Knee to Chest Two sets / six reps / 30-second rest between sets
- Shoulder Stretch Two sets / eight reps / 30 seconds rest
- Heel-To-Toe Walk Two sets / eight reps / 30 seconds rest
- Knee To Chest Pose Two sets / Four reps each leg / 30 seconds rest
- Head and Thumb Sync Two sets / ten reps each arm / 30 seconds rest

Week 3: Sitting Strong, Core Fitness, Verti-Go Away

Day 1 Routine

- Overhead Side Stretch Two sets / eight reps / 30-second rest between sets
- Soleus Stretch Two sets / four reps / 30-second rest between sets
- Triceps Stretch Two sets / eight reps / 30 seconds rest
- Seated Calf Raises Three sets / ten reps / 30 seconds rest
- Wood Chops Two sets / eight reps (4 each side) / 30 seconds rest
- Epley Maneuver Two sets / three reps each side / 30 seconds rest

Day 2 Routine

- Seated Knee to Chest Two sets / six reps / 30-second rest between sets
- Hamstring Stretch Two sets / six reps / 30-second rest between sets
- Soleus Stretch Two sets / four reps / 30 seconds rest
- Sit to Stand Two sets / ten reps 20 / 30 seconds rest
- Dead Bug Two sets / four reps each leg / 30 seconds rest
- Foster Maneuver Two sets / four reps / 30 seconds rest

Day 3 Routine

- Overhead Side Stretch Stretch Two sets / eight reps / 30-second rest between sets
- Soleus Stretch Two sets / four reps / 30-second rest between sets
- Shoulder Stretch Two sets / eight reps / 30 seconds rest
- Seated Marches Three sets / ten reps / 30 seconds rest
- Flamingo Stand Two sets / Ten seconds per leg / 30 seconds rest
- Brandt Daroff Exercise Two sets / 20 second reps / 30 seconds rest

Week 4: Standing Strong, Floor Work, Watch Your Step

Day 1 Routine

- Hamstring Stretch Two sets / six reps / 30-second rest between sets
- Standing Quad Stretch Two sets / eight reps / 30-second rest between sets
- Overhead Side Stretch Two sets / eight reps / 30 seconds rest
- Straight Leg Raises to The Back Two sets / four raises per leg / 30 seconds rest
- Clam Shells Three sets / eight reps / 30 seconds rest
- Side Step Claps Two sets / eight reps / 30 seconds rest

Day 2 Routine

- Seated Knee To Chest Two sets / six reps / 30-second rest between sets
- Soleus Stretch Two sets / four reps / 30-second rest between sets

- Shoulder Stretch Two sets / eight reps / 30 seconds rest
- Weight Shifts Two sets / 30 seconds right, 30 Seconds left / 30 seconds rest
- Side Hip Raises Two sets / five reps left, five reps right / 30 seconds rest
- Standing March with Arm movement Three sets / 12 reps / 30 seconds rest

Day 3 Routine

- Hamstring Stretch Two sets / six reps / 30-second rest between sets
- Soleus Stretch Two sets / four reps / 30-second rest between sets
- Overhead Side Stretch Two sets / eight reps / 30 seconds rest
- Alternate Leg In & Out Two sets / six reps per leg / 30 seconds rest
- Trunk Rotations Two sets / six reps per leg / 30 seconds rest
- Balance Steps Two sets / 20 steps / 30 seconds rest

CONCLUSION

Every one of us wants to live a happy and healthy life. But certain conditions simply can't be avoided, such as aging. It comes with its pros and mostly the cons. Many people start to feel weak and unstable. Many people begin facing balance issues in old age. This book has covered the exercises to regain the lost balance. Each exercise has been discussed with step-by-step instructions.

The goal of balance exercises is to improve overall body stability and coordination. When walking, biking, climbing stairs, or dancing, balance helps you stay upright. Even as you get older, it's critical to do exercises that improve your balance. It is easier to avoid injuries if you have a good balance. Because older people are more vulnerable to accidents involving slips and falls, it's critical to maintain your balance as you age.

The exercises discussed in the book are designed to help you maintain your body's natural alignment. Because your muscles and bones naturally wear down as you age, performing these exercises regularly can help you maintain your current lifestyle. You can do these exercises at home with items you already have.

It's never too late to start an exercise routine or improve the one you already have. Walking, chair yoga and tai chi are all excellent ways to improve your balance in addition to these exercises. Make it a point to engage in physical activity every day, even if it is only for a few minutes. You'll be more likely to stick to your routine if you do it this way.

Include strength training, cardio, stretching in your routine, and balance exercises. Make sure you eat a well-balanced diet that will help you maintain a healthy weight for your body type. Most importantly, remember to have fun while making these positive changes to your life.

SCAN ME FOR VIDEO

THANK YOU FOR READING!

https://www.amazon.com/review/create-review?&asin=B0C2B2JQ9P

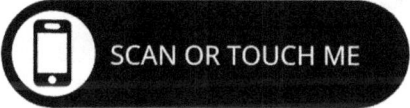

Use QR code above to leave honest feedback

SAFETY CONSIDERATION

Balance exercises are essential for older adults, but they must be done with caution. Ensure you have something nearby to help you maintain your balance, such as a chair, a wall, or another person. Take frequent breaks and don't attempt to accomplish too much at once. If you have any concerns about beginning a new balance program or if these exercises cause you any pain, consult your doctor before continuing.

Warm up for a few minutes before you begin your workout. Stretch for another 5 minutes after you've finished exercising. Consult your doctor in case of emergency or if your symptoms are worsening.

REFERENCES

List of references

Lin, H. W., & Bhattacharyya, N. (2012). Balance disorders in the elderly: epidemiology and functional impact. The Laryngoscope, 122(8), 1858-1861.

Berg, R. L., & Cassells, J. S. (1992). Falls in older persons: risk factors and prevention. In The second fifty years: Promoting health and preventing disability. National Academies Press (US).

Seguin, R., & Nelson, M. E. (2003). The benefits of strength training for older adults. American journal of preventive medicine, 25(3), 141-149.

Volpi, E., Nazemi, R., & Fujita, S. (2004). Muscle tissue changes with aging. Current opinion in clinical nutrition and metabolic care, 7(4), 405.

Centers for Disease Control and Prevention. (2017). Depression is Not a Normal Part of Growing Older. Division of Population Health, updates January 31, 2017.

Hafström, A., Malmström, E. M., Terdèn, J., Fransson, P. A., & Magnusson, M. (2016). Improved balance confidence and stability for elderly after 6 weeks of a multimodal self-administered balance-enhancing exercise program: a randomized single-arm crossover study. Gerontology and geriatric medicine, 2, 2333721416644149.

9 simple and important stretching exercises for seniors. https://iorapri-marycare.com/blog/stretching-exercises-for-seniors/

How to become more flexible and tips to try. https://www.trustedhealth-products.com/blogs/natural-health-news/how-to-become-more-flexi-ble-stretching-exercises-and-tips-to-try

7 total body stretches for older adults by Divya 2022, https://www.s-portskeeda.com/health-and-fitness/7-best-total-body-stretches-older-adults

https://fitnessconnection.com/featured/be-thankful-for-fitness/

What is the alternating superman exercise? Tips, Technique, Correct Form, Benefits, and Common Mistakes. By Divya, 2022. https://www.s-portskeeda.com/health-and-fitness/what-alternating-superman-exer-cise-tips-technique-correct-form